HOW TO BUY
TECHNOLOGY

NG9-1-1 Recording and Dispatch Improvement

JOE MOSED

DSS CORPORATION / EQUATURE

How to Buy Technology:

NG9-1-1 Recording and Dispatch Improvement

First Edition.

ISBN 13 Digit: 978-1-933598-68-0

Published by Johnson & Hunter, Inc.

Trademarks

For Joe Mosed Sr., Thank you for making me the 3rd option

Contents

Acknowledgement

Putting a book together is a team effort. Wanting to write a book and actually doing it are two very different things. There is no way I could have done this without the support of my family. I would also like to thank the stakeholders of DSS Corporation including our team members, partners and most of all our customers. Our customers are in the life saving business and we understand that Seconds Save Lives.

March 8, 2012
Detroit, Michigan

Introduction

I am writing this introduction four days after my twin girls were born. The girls, to give you a play-by-play, are huge. Their combined weight averages that of the offensive line for Michigan State's football team. Zoey comes in at a bulky three pounds nine ounces and Brooklyn makes her debut at an astonishing four pounds ten ounces.

Rushing back and forth from the hospital and NICU was a whirlwind of activity. Fortunately, for me, Beaverton Police Officer Anderson understood. He has twins—which was the only reason he let me off with a warning. (Talking on the phone, speeding, and not having insurance information are not recommended.) At first, I was not sure how he knew to ask if I had twins, then I realized I was wearing two hospital wristbands. I know, you think I came up with a cheesy story to get out of the ticket. I did not. Officer Anderson noticed the bands and asked. The good news is he saved me over $700 in fees. It pays to have something in common.

New parents are typically clueless until reality sets in. You can read books, watch videos, and talk to other parents, but when it comes right down to it you do not understand what it is like to have children until you walk the path. As a dad, I wonder:

- What if something happens to one of the girls?
- What do I do if there is an issue with one of the girls?

- What if my wife freaks out because Zoey has another choking scare?

As much as I hope these things never happen to anyone, the reality is these situations and others occur every day.

What does this have to do with NG9-1-1 Recording and Dispatch Improvement? As a father, I can tell you it has *everything* to do with dispatch improvement. When there is a life-threatening issue, who do people call? 9-1-1. Dispatchers have the power to save lives. Every second counts in an emergency situation. Seconds Save Lives.

Currently, people cannot send text messages, videos, or pictures to Dispatch Centers. This is a big deal because this additional data would save seconds and offer better response times for first responders. This is where NG9-1-1 (Next Generation 9-1-1) will have the greatest impact. Another issue is that young people text far more than they talk on the phone. Not being able to text 9-1-1 is a monster disconnect that NG9-1-1 will remedy.

Dispatch improvement is a critical component because the amount of data that comes at dispatchers will increase by at least three times. If the proper tools are not in place, the training and learning will be under par which is not acceptable when lives are on the line.

Dispatchers live and breathe stress every day which yields high turnover and burnout rates. This is a problem for Dispatch Center team leads and directors because they must constantly seek and train new people.

One goal of this book is to educate Dispatch Center personnel on NG9-1-1 Recording and Dispatch Improvement. Your feedback is encouraged because it is my goal to always improve and drive relevant content to our user community.

Please contact me directly with any questions, comments, and suggestions (good or bad) as this book will continue to live and evolve on our blog.

Joe Mosed
President, DSS Corporation
(866) 377-2677

1

Selling

Selling to the government is not easy. If I had any sense, I would have exited the business. There are much easier ways to make a living. Flowing through government bureaucracy and long sales cycles can be discouraging. From a profit-and-revenue-generation standpoint, there are more lucrative and faster markets to target. I bring this up to illustrate the point that to be in the government space, you need to have an affinity for the market. Remember that Dispatch Centers and first responders are responsible for saving lives. This is a much bigger purpose than profit. (Profit is not bad. Profit is required for future R&D and other innovations that customers expect.)

When we ponder the dilemma of the buyer-seller dance, we need to understand that people want to buy.

Good buyers understand what they want. In the dispatch field, you are working with the following cast of characters: the board, management, dispatch supervisors, dispatch team leads, dispatchers, and IT. You need to satisfy all of their needs and select the right solution. And you have to be accountable to taxpayers because you are spending tax dollars. Citizen satisfaction and excellent public safety are the required end result. The goal is to find a balance between Great Service, Great Quality, and Great Pricing.

Great service, great quality, and great pricing are oxymoronic. You need to understand you can only have two; no company can provide all three. Let me give you some examples to cement this point.

1. **McDonald's** – McDonald's has mastered great pricing and great service but NOT great quality. You don't take your better half on a romantic date to McDonald's.

2. **Costco** - Costco has mastered great pricing and great quality. They have excellent products and their pricing is perfect for bulk buyers. They do NOT have great service. You need to stand in long lines and bring your own boxes or use theirs to box up your purchases. You also have limited payment options. Great Service is not one of their staples.

3. **Apple** – Apple has mastered Great Quality and Great Service. Their products are elegant and high quality. They provide outstanding service. When you walk into an Apple store, they have the Genius bar and will help you with anything. There is no traditional cashier and you can stay as long as you like. Apple does NOT have great pricing. Their pricing is much higher than competing brands.

You need to understand what your Dispatch Center's priorities are before selling the NG9-1-1 Recording and Dispatch Improvement.

Buyers (Communication Director, 911 Director, etc.) need to understand the needs of all stakeholders. When purchasing a recording system, the stakeholders are: the board, dispatchers, team leads, IT, and the agency as a whole. The recording platform needs to consist of Great Quality and Great Service. Pricing is secondary. Remember, these solutions act as insurance. When the floods come, you want to make sure you are covered. Buying these solutions based on price is a mistake that you might not be able to recover from.

Here are the initial questions you ask when starting your buying process. To download a full questionnaire, visit
http://www.dispatchimprovement.com/book/buying-questions.aspx

1. What are the three biggest concerns you need to address with the recording system?

2. How much time do you spend using the system now? Doing what?

3. How often do you receive Freedom of Information Requests (FOIA) from the public?

4. How long do these take to fulfill? Can it be improved?

5. How do you share information with your District Attorney's (DA) office?

6. How many requests do you receive weekly from the DA's office?

7. How long does it take to fulfill the requests from the DA's office?

Understanding your current landscape is critical to acquire the right recording system and to create the best partnership. Begin with the end in mind.

When it comes to purchasing a recording system, the three most important needs to consider are Simplicity, Reliability, and Speed. All concerns fall into these three areas. Here are some examples to illustrate my point:

1. **Speed** – When there is a service issue, how fast is it resolved? Real-time access. Seconds save lives so the system cannot be slow. Dispatchers need Live Recall to verify addresses and other lifesaving information.

2. **Simplicity** – Dispatch Center personnel have diverse skill sets. The platform has to be easy to use or users will not adopt it. Think about this: how much formal training have you had using Google? How easy is it to do business with your new partner? Say no to voicemail jail☺. This is especially critical in a crisis situation.

3. **Reliability** – The system needs to be on 24/7/365. Your recording partner needs to be passionate about this because Dispatch Centers depend on it. How reliable is the service after the implementation? This is critical because if it is a hit-and-run, you will be stuck with the system and a marginal vendor.

I can tell you, we have never received a phone call from agencies wishing they would have saved the extra 15 percent. All of the frustrations revolve around Simplicity, Reliability, and Speed. None of them revolve around price. To further illustrate this fact, let's chat about Commodity Buying vs. Solution Buying.

Commodity Buying vs. Solution Buying

In the Dispatch Center commodities are items like paper, office supplies, and utilities. Solution buying typically involves equipment that is kept for several years and used by many people. Things like the radio system, 911 call premise equipment, CAD, and the recording system. These require more thought and planning before agencies buy. Solution buying is a team effort because there are several casts of characters that use the systems once they are installed.

Copycat Buying

Before purchasing dispatch recording equipment, directors want to know what others are using. This is social proof that the vendor selection is correct. It is basically copycat buying and can be very effective. "If the agency next door purchased from XYZ, then I should, too" is the mantra. Before you blindly follow copycat buying, you need to consider a few points.

What are the goals of your Dispatch Center? When looking at other agencies, are their goals the same as yours? Are they world-class in their service delivery? Are they committed to Dispatch Improvement and continuous learning so they can provide first responders and citizens with the best service possible? If this is NOT the case, I suggest you rethink copying their purchasing decisions.

I realize this may sound harsh, but to be great, you must imitate greatness. It is still prudent to find out what your neighbors are buying so you are comfortable in your decision—but it is recommended that you define greatness for your center and emulate other great centers. This will take work, but is worth it. Emulating greatness will also allow your center to grow if you are in areas of consolidation. Right now, consolidating Dispatch Centers for economies of scale is prevalent around the country. If you are bidding to dispatch for other agencies, those agencies want to make sure you can do it better than they can.

Cast of Characters

Let's dive into the nuts and bolts of the Next Generation 911 recording system. To avoid putting you to sleep, the heavy-duty technical data is in the appendices.

Dispatcher – Dispatchers are front-line gurus and masters at multi-tasking. Good dispatchers are worth their weight in gold because they do a job that 90 percent of the population cannot. I have great respect for them and you should, too. When one of your family members is in trouble, it is a dispatcher that will save him or her. Remember – Seconds Save Lives. Dispatchers need two basic functionalities from the recording system: real-time access to their calls/NG data and the ability to tag that information EASILY. This is critically important because when there is an issue it needs to be found right away. Dispatchers will need additional training when NG911 is deployed because the content coming at them is three times what it is today. Remember, people twenty-five years and younger text more than they talk.

Dispatch Supervisor – These wonderful people are responsible for a ton of things, including training and quality review. The recording platform is critical for this function. Unfortunately several agencies perform quality reviews either ad hoc or manually. There are two reasons to automate this function: time and money. Automated quality assessment is critical for dispatch personnel to improve. With budgets slashed, people achieve more work with less help. The quality portion of the recording system needs to be automated and easy. These are the two main uses for dispatch supervisors.

Certified Training Officer– Some agencies have CTO's (Certified Training Officers). These people are responsible for the training content and the delivery of the training. Another big component is scheduling, allocating resources along with the correct dispatching coverage. This is critical and becomes a major task in large centers. The recording platform plays a key role in content retrieval and training to accomplish the goals set by the Certified Training Officer.

Records – Historical search for incident discovery for court and FOIA requests are part of Records. The requirements for the recording system are extensive. The major requirements include: 100 percent content search, tagging, and data sharing. What this means is that records personnel should be able to type in a "word or phrase" and find the relevant interaction as if conducting a Google search. In the old days, records personnel would go to the CAD system, look at the CAD number, and pull the date and time. With that information, they would then go to the recording system and search by time and date. Now, the fun begins. After they pulled back 300 calls, they would listen to them to see which ones pertained to the incident. Agencies no longer have time for this nonsense.

The second critical feature is the ability to type in any search like CAD Number, Radio ID, address, and call type along with a spoken word and find exactly what you want— INSTANTLY.

First Responders – Seconds Save Lives. First Responders need access to emergency information as it is happening. Call and incident information sharing is required on any device. Recording platforms need to provide information instantly on a Mobile Data Terminal, Android Tablet, iPad, iPhone, or Android phone. Real-time data is critical when lives are on the line.

Directors – Directors need to keep the user base happy. Managing a Dispatch Center can be like herding cats all day. Directors serve many masters. As an example, we see service centers that dispatch fourteen fire posts, eighteen police departments, and four ambulance companies. With consolidation efforts in the works, this type of coverage is becoming commonplace around the country. In addition, Directors serve the general public, county commissioners, and state offices. The last thing a director needs is vendor headaches. This is where vendors need to put their money where their mouth is. Basically the recording system needs to work as stated. True partners guarantee this in writing. I will discuss protecting yourself and obtaining written guarantees later.

The Board – The board consists of elected officials who deal with agency business. They are an interface between tax dollars and the public. Typically, boards trust their directors and will support the directors' decisions. Regardless, it is the board's job to make sure the agency, citizens, and taxpayers are all taken care of and represented. Understanding these objectives will have agencies acquire the solutions they want and need to get the job done. Most of the time, the board wants to help in these endeavors. When a solution is not the low bid, the board needs a valid understanding of why the selection was made. Remember, they are the front line to the taxpayers and when asked, they need to respond intelligently.

Information Technology (IT) – The beloved IT department is crucial because it keeps things working. IT personnel want solutions that work and meld into their environment. All of the systems need to talk with each other and play nice together. Some of the biggest headaches IT departments face are with users' computers. The servers in the back room (that nobody sees) typically run smoothly because IT controls them. User computers can be different for one main reason: USERS. In terms of the recording system, reliability is critical but there are several other things that IT people want. The two main ones are browser-based user interface and security. The last thing IT wants is to install software on hundreds of user's computers. If a system uses a browser, this is not necessary. Also, IT spends a lot of time setting up network security and the recorder needs to adhere to it. (I will profile the technical jargon in a separate section so you don't fall asleep.)

Selling the Board

Great leaders know they need to influence people for positive outcomes. Positional leadership is the lowest rung of the leadership ladder, i.e., just because you are the boss does not mean you are an effective leader. People will do the bare minimum if they work for an ineffective leader. Great leaders understand the nuances of influence and make it a lifelong pursuit to master it.

There are six core behaviors that affect sales persuasion. These are great concepts and they are based on research. (For more information read the book *Influence* by Dr. Robert Cialdini.)

1. **Reciprocation**

According to Emerson's law of compensation, if you want more then give more. When you give something to somebody, they feel indebted and compelled to give back. This is backed up by research. Dr. Cialdini did a study of waiters/waitresses and found that when they gave mints to their customers their tips increased. He also found that when they came back to the table and gave each patron an additional mint their tips increased by 23 percent. There are countless studies showing the power of reciprocation.

How does this apply to dispatch centers and the board? When you decide that you want a particular solution and it is not the lowest price, then you need to let the board know before the public meetings. Give the directors a simple report that shows why it makes sense to go this way. Show them the value from their point of view and they will reward you with providing the tools you need to continue saving lives.

2. **Commitment / Consistency**

When people say something or make a decision, they need to stand by it. Their actions need to follow their words. When people do not do this, then they are seen as untrustworthy. Toy stores mastered this concept. In January and February sales were low because parents shopped in December. The toy stores fixed this problem by using the power of commitment and consistency. Toy manufacturers start to advertise the hot, new item before Christmas and all the kids want the new whiz-bang toy. During the holiday shopping season, the manufacturers limit the supply of the toy. Then, in January and February, stocks are replenished and parents return to the toy store to purchase little Johnny his PROMISED toy. When parents promise their kids a particular toy they feel obligated to deliver even though Christmas is past. So, how is this applicable to selling the board? Typically, boards are committed to citizen satisfaction and the public. To stand behind that commitment, the board needs to provide Dispatch Centers the right tools to provide the BEST service to its citizens. These need to be provided even if the price is not the lowest. Show the board why the solution you want provides better service based on their commitment and you will get what you want.

3. Social Proof

Social Proof is the icing on the cake. Basically, people want to be unique but they also want to know that the item they buy works. Social Proof gives them that comfort. There is a saying in the tech world that "nobody was ever fired for buying IBM." This is classic social proof. To provide your board with social proof make sure your vendor partner provided you with good, solid references.

4. Liking

In a nut shell, people like to buy from people like them. When you are selling to your board, you need to understand their point of view. When you do, they will appreciate it and reward you with the best tools to do your job. Remember:

"People don't care what you know until they know how much you care."

5. Authority

People like to be validated by authority figures. Think about this. Your best friend can give advice for you to lose weight. You take it with a grain of salt. When your doctor says you have to lose weight or you will die, you end up losing the weight. The doctor had more authority than your best friend. To utilize this in your system purchase, look for the vendor's expertise as it relates to NG9-1-1. Do they participate in all the events? Do they chair committees and write specification for organizations like APCO (Association of Public Safety Communications Officials) and NENA (National Emergency Number Association)?

6. Scarcity

Avoiding scarcity is a primal function and is at the bottom of Dr. Abraham Maslow's hierarchy of needs. It is why people line up at the Apple store to purchase the next generation iPhone. It is why limited-quantity cars sell for a premium. The strongest example I can give you on scarcity involves investing in the stock market. Everybody logically knows that you should buy low and sell high. Regardless of this fact, most people do the exact opposite: they sell when the stock is tanking because they feel the SCARCITY effect on their money. Likewise, they buy when others are buying because they feel the SCARCITY of the opportunity slipping away. This strong emotional behavior trumps logic every time. And it is applicable when selling to the board because having a unique feature or better public service is a competitive advantage for the community. Remember people make decisions to move into a community based on public safety.

Vendor Business Models

When purchasing new programs and equipment for your Dispatch Center, you need to understand the business models of your partners. This is important because it will dictate 50 percent of the relationship. If you view this relationship like a marriage, then you want to be educated before you take the plunge. Divorce rate is above 50 percent and you don't want to end up there with the recorder purchase decision.

1. **Large, publically traded vendors** – This business model provides a level of safety for agencies because these vendors "may" have a strong balance sheet and cash position. This means that they are not going anywhere anytime soon. Some of the positives:

    i.   Strong financials: need to verify and look at their debt.

    ii. Global in nature.

    iii. Multiple markets: security, financial, call centers, and public safety.

   These are good benefits if they have a strong commitment to Public Safety. Some potential drawbacks:

    i.   Headquartered Overseas: Manufactured overseas (American jobs).

    ii. Distribution Model has many layers: overseas headquarters, stateside regional offices, resellers, then your Dispatch Center.

iii. Support Model has many layers: overseas headquarters for development, stateside sales office, then reseller technicians for minor support or replacements.

iv. Reporting Requirements: Wall Street demands short-term gains; this is a problem if management is only focused on the next quarter. This can provide issues as we saw with big banks, Enron, and WorldCom.

In summary, large, publically traded vendors offer financial stability which can be a major positive.

2. **Resellers** – These organizations are customer-focused. In the recording market, most of these organizations are small and typically the principal is the main sales contact. This is good for Dispatch Centers because response is usually good. Some positive highlights:

i. Very responsive: These organizations understand that customer service is critical for their survival.

ii. Flexible: These organizations are typically easy to do business with and will not make you jump through a ton of hoops to get your objectives accomplished.

iii. Variety: These organizations sell multiple recorders and offer a commodity-based decision to their customers, i.e., you select the features you want.

Some drawbacks to this business model are:

    i.   Resellers cannot bind the manufacturer. If promises on functionality or enhancements are made by the reseller, the manufacturer is not required to fulfill the promises.

    ii. Limited resources: Organizations that sell multiple products are not experts on any of the products. Thus, for major technical support, the manufacturer has to take over.

    iii. Product turnover: You buy recorder A and five years later you are being sold recorder B. This may have worked in the past but is no longer valid because of data retention, storage, and other factors affecting NG9-1-1.

In summary, the reseller model has some benefits and was a critical model in the 1980s and 1990s for selling proprietary recorders.

3. **Direct Manufacturers** – These businesses have real advantages today for Dispatch Centers; they are:

    i.   One organization owns the relationship. Direct manufacturers make, sell, train, and support the platform. This avoids finger-pointing and gives agencies more control of the relationship.

    ii. Platform enhancements are faster because direct manufacturers deal directly with the end users. Remember agencies are responsible for product enhancements and new features.

Things don't get lost in translation because of the direct relationship.

iii. Support: This is critical because level 1 to level 3 development support are handled directly by the manufacturer. This dramatically shortens support response times and case resolution times.

iv. Expertise: Direct manufacturers are experts on both their recording solution and the markets they serve.

The negatives of this model are:

i. Social Proof: You may have never heard of the manufacturer since this is a newer model for this market. Comfort levels are not yet established.

ii. Most recorder purchases in the past were from resellers; entering into a new relationship is uncomfortable for some agencies. This is another variant of social proof.

In summary, agencies might be hesitant with change but this business model has some positive attributes and will most likely be the wave of the future.

From Ad Hoc Quality to Dispatch Improvement

Dispatching and running Dispatch Centers is hard work. The stress levels and burnout rates run high. To mitigate this, agencies are implementing dispatch-improvement programs.

The recording platform provides not only real-time access but also an archival repository for training. Some agencies listen to archived calls and then fill out paper forms. These forms are shared with the dispatcher and improvements are suggested. However, with budget cuts and time constraints, training in this fashion is no longer valid because it makes historical trending and improvement tracking excessively difficult.

Dispatch-improvement platforms are automated and provide agencies with relevant trending and historical data. Also, the information is available to dispatchers for periodic review and skill set training based on best practices.

Effective dispatch-improvement tools consist of the following modules:

1. **Assessment Forms.** The NG recorder needs to have the ability to create assessment forms in an easy-to-use method with no programming involved. The forms must be flexible and support any question type.

2. Screen Capture. Interactions are paired up with the dispatchers' screens so supervisors get the full picture of what happened.

3. 100 percent Content Search. This is critical for automating calls so that only calls that matter get assessed by supervisors. As an example, you can assess all calls that contain the phrase "**shots fired**" and have them delivered to your supervisor instantly.

4. Automated Review. This saves time and increases dispatch improvement by automating the selection and delivery method for supervisors.

5. Unlimited Reviews. Once assessments are completed, you want to share them with dispatchers and allow them to make comments and perform self-review. This is an effective way to start training-dialogue and remove subjectivity. Collaboration between supervisors and dispatchers is critical for true dispatch improvement.

2

911 Recording

Traditional 911 recording is what you are used to. The platform records radio, 911, and telephone traffic and has a user interface to access that data. Search is basically 5 percent of the repository, meaning you can search on Time/Date, Channel, and other simple criteria like caller phone number and ANI/ALI (address and number location). This is very basic.

A quick history of the recording market shows there were two major players in the recording space. In the 1950s, Dictaphone and Magnasync made Open Reel recording systems.

These contraptions basically recorded one day's worth of information on a large tape the size of a serving platter. These tapes sold for about $150 each. Most agencies would keep thirty days' worth of recording because the storage was so expensive. Since searching and finding information was a nightmare on these recorders, they sat in the back room with little value other than insurance.

In 1992, two manufacturers changed the landscape with the introduction of VHS-based recording. They were TEAC and

Racal. These recorders could fit on a desk and the tapes were only $10 each. Agencies flocked to the new technology because it was easier to use, required less space which allowed them to keep more data. The pricing was obviously much more attractive as well.

After VHS technology came the first digital recorders. These systems recorded to DAT tape and introduced the concept of channel hours, meaning that the tape no longer moved continuously. With digital, the silence time was able to be compressed and storage increased. The Dictaphone 9800 took the field by storm. This product was actually made by Eventide. The benefits to the agency were the following: more storage, easier playback, and less media management.

One drawback of the DAT tape format, however, was that the search time on archived media was still slow. TEAC introduced optical disk technology and took the market by storm with their CR500 model. This machine allowed almost instant access to older recordings, which was unheard of in the market.

Optical disk technology then morphed into DVD technology, along with network-based recording systems.

Today recording systems are much more advanced with unlimited storage, unlimited users, and more functionality. Recorders purchased today need to be NG9-1-1 ready as well.

Now let's look at NG9-1-1 recording.

NG9-1-1 Recording

NG9-1-1 Recording opens up all media types beyond voice. Currently, if you are hiding in a closet and text **HELP!** to

911, Dispatch does not receive the text. This is a serious problem because of the proliferation of cell phones, smart phones, and smart devices. The Internet has been around for a long time and people deserve NG9-1-1 capabilities today.

Next Generation 9-1-1 allows for voice, pictures, video, telematics (car crash data), and other data to be received by the Dispatch Center.

The goal is to provide better citizen response and share this data with first responders. Remember, Seconds Save Lives. Anything that comes into a Dispatch Center needs to be recorded or logged, hence NG9-1-1 recording.

Techy Jargon

NG9-1-1 has several components including data routing, networks, and interoperability. NG9-1-1recorders need to have three core components. The first is component is called **SIP Bridge recording**. SIP is a protocol that all communications will travel. This is similar to voice-over IP but includes any message type. SIP by definition is Session Initiation Protocol. The bridged recording connects to the ESInet which is the network that will carry all the NG data and records the information. One critical component of this is that the recorder can exist anywhere on the network. This is important for agencies looking to share services and save money. (This is similar in concept to cloud computing and shared services.)

The second mandatory component is the **Logging Service**. The logging service is the piece that records all the metadata associated with the interaction. One key difference under NG9-1-1 is that agencies can transfer interactions and all of the data stays intact. This does not happen today. If there is a high-speed chase crossing agency boundaries and the call is transferred, all the associated data is lost. This is eliminated with NG9-1-1 and the Logging Service acts as the archiving piece of all the data.

The third core mandatory component is **Interoperability**. NG9-1-1 recorders are required to share the data they capture in a NON-PROPRIETARY method. This is done through REAL TIME STREAMING PROTOCOL (RTSP). Basically this means that any NG equipment on the network, along with authorized users, can obtain information in a standard way. This is a paradigm shift because interoperability is required.

Why is Interoperability Important?

What is interoperability? *Interoperability* means that systems need to be able to talk with each other. Currently, 911 systems speak their own languages. There are systems that speak English, German, Chinese, and Spanish and they don't understand each other. NG9-1-1 requires manufacturers to interoperate and speak the same language.

This can get technical; if you want more details, you can check out the free download at
http://www.dispatchimprovement.com/book/911-briefing.aspx

To sum up, interoperability allows different systems to communicate seamlessly and to understand each other. This is important because it saves agencies from having to spend a ton of money on custom one-off integrations. Additional benefits of interoperability are data sharing, administration, vendor choice, and cost savings.

Guarantees

Why are guarantees important? I realize this seems like a stupid question, but I am shocked by how many agencies don't get guarantees in writing. The partner you choose should give this to you WITHOUT you having to ask for it. Guarantees offer agencies buyer protection. The crafting of a good guarantee allows the Dispatch Center to return the equipment for non-performance. True partners will guarantee even more than the purchase price. This is a reflection of the value of the buyer's time. Having a 110 percent guarantee on a solution is like having an ace up your sleeve. This is designed to make buyers comfortable and to eliminate all buyer risk. To guarantee system performance or particular functionality requires the written guarantee to be from the manufacturer of the equipment. If you are dealing with a reseller organization then they need to provide this guarantee in writing from the manufacturer. A sample of our guarantee is included in Appendix B.

Next Generation 9-1-1 is the framework for Dispatch Centers to accept all methods of communications, including text, chat, video, pictures, and voice. Other components include sensor data, vehicle telematics, and alarm data. (Vehicle telematics is the data that OnStar uses. In an accident, the severity level and other information is collected and sent to the OnStar service center.)

You might wonder why all types of communications aren't accepted. After all, the Internet has been around since the 1960s and in the mainstream since the early 1990s.

When 911 centers provide service, the information must be instantly available. Remember Seconds Save Lives. As you know, you can send a text or an email to someone and it might get there in two seconds or thirty minutes. This disparity is unacceptable to 911 Dispatch Centers. Because of the non-guarantee of service provided by current infrastructure, agencies need to build high-availability networks. Yes, these networks use Internet protocols and current technologies—but the engineering and priority routing is different.

The Emergency Services Internetwork (ESInet) is the plumbing and backbone of all NG9-1-1 systems. This infrastructure can exist anywhere from an individual PSAP (Public Safety Answering Point), county, multiple counties, statewide, and/or nationwide. DSS has found that each area of the country is unique on how it rolls out its ESInet but the plumbing is the same regardless if it is regional or statewide. The constraints at this level are differentiated by funding, and local and state government mandates. The new NG9-1-1 infrastructure also has to bridge current networks and support them all. Examples of existing networks include Public Access IP networks, public switched telephone networks (landline, satellite, and cellular) as well as public safety radio networks.

The diagram below sums up in a basic way NG9-1-1 as a whole. Here is an example of how it works: Let's suppose there is a major car accident. People call 911 from their smart phones and they also send pictures and video of the crash from these devices. If there are traffic cameras in the area, that footage can also be sent to the Dispatch Center. This information is accepted by dispatch and used to send the appropriate first responders (like police, fire and EMS). If the Dispatch Center is authorized to take EMD calls, medical advice will also be communicated. ... And, here is where the power of NG9-1-1 comes into play. The visual and vehicle telematics data can be shared with the first responders while they are en route. Remember SECONDS SAVE LIVES. This simple change will save lives and give first responders better data before they even reach the destination. One caveat: any dispatcher, director, or other public safety professional knows that the single biggest imperative is to GET TO THE RIGHT LOCATION. For centers that dispatch for large geographic areas, this is absolutely critical. The last thing you want to do is dispatch to 123 Main Street in Rochester if is 123 Main Street in Birmingham. (Side Note: I was shadowing in a Dispatch Center and this problem came up. There was an incident with a child and the location was incorrect. The responders went to the right street number in the WRONG city. Unfortunately, they were too late. You can see why dispatch personnel have such high levels of stress. Everybody reading this book needs to thank a dispatcher. These men and women have an unbelievably hard job and if there is any technology, process, or procedure that can help them, we need to give it to them.)

CORRECT INFORMATION AT THE CORRECT TIME SAVES LIVES. With NG9-1-1, you can see the pictures and the location on your computer screen. This will immensely help reduce location-based issues.

All the data (pictures, video, etc.) can now be pushed out and shared to the first responders. While en route, they can prepare for what is needed at the scene because THEY CAN SEE IT beforehand. This is huge and will improve the landscape for all public safety.

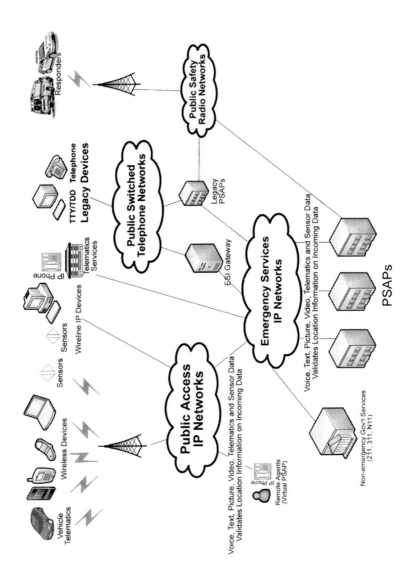

All of the data in the above illustration must be recorded or logged. Before I get into those details, let's dive into the interoperability component of NG9-1-1. As you can see from the basic description of NG9-1-1 infrastructure, there are several components and pieces. (If you were to explore the bits and bytes of this, you would be thumbing through thousands of pages of technical data.) Since I want you to read this book, I will not include that information here. Instead, you can find more information in Appendix A.

Interoperability is imperative for the various components to seamlessly work together. Open standards and nonproprietary methods are employed. The good news is the NG initiative requires interoperability. Vendors who want to play in this field must code and make their solutions to the open standards defined by the NG9-1-1 standards. The key components of interoperability are:

1. NG Standards allow systems from different vendors to interoperate "right out of the box."

2. Major PSAP (Public Safety Answering Point) systems can be anywhere on the network and so can personnel.

3. NG allows you to easily consolidate and share systems as "services" with other jurisdictions.

4. This all adds up to better functionality at lower costs because costs can be shared and set up as "services."

NG9-1-1 Recording

The three main components of NG9-1-1 recording are: SIP Recording, the Logging Service, and RTSP data sharing. These are all nonproprietary and coded so any vendor can meet the specifications outlined by the NG committees.

The best way to understand the logging service is to look at the diagram on the next page.

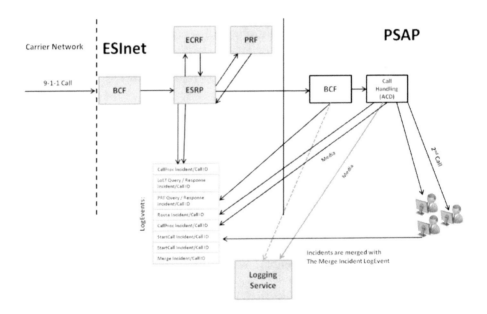

1. **The Logging Service** - This diagram represents a 9-1-1 call in the NG9-1-1 environment. Without going into a full technical description of the diagram, I simply want you to take away two important points:

a. Under NG9-1-1 all data that moves from one agency to the next agency stays intact. This is significant because, today, if a call is transferred from agency A to agency B, all the ANI/ALI and other location-based data is lost and agency B does not see it.

b. Under NG9-1-1 there is additional relevant data that is associated with the calls (interactions) and all of that data needs to be logged.

The logging service is a new component for NG9-1-1 recording. Its purpose is to log all of the data that is associated with NG9-1-1 interactions over the ESInet. These interactions can be associated with the calls, but do not have to be. ESInet's cannot go live until they have a logging service attached. This piece is a critical component of NG9-1-1 recording.

The diagram below is a visual of an NG9-1-1 recording system. The three components are highlighted in blue. The LogEvents logging service on the bottom left is a visual display of that capability to log all the interactions data.

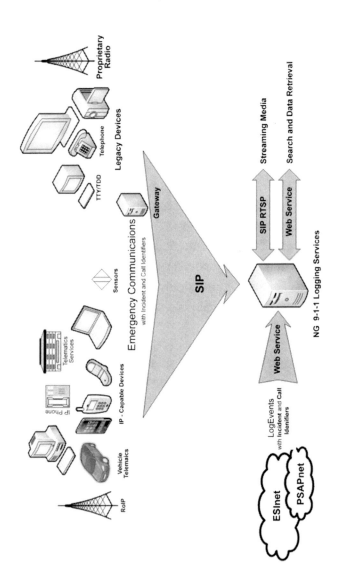

All of the interactions (calls, pictures, videos, and NG data) travel over the ESInet using the SIP protocol. This protocol is designed to carry messaging data and is an open standard. SIP stands for Session Initiation Protocol and was popularized in the traditional VoIP (Voice over Internet Protocol) world. The protocol can carry any message type and is used extensively in NG9-1-1.

There are two ways to record this information; any vendor you choose to partner with should support both.

2. **SIP SPAN** – A port on the network is dedicated to the recording system and all traffic is mirrored to that port. The recorder sniffs the mirrored traffic and records it accordingly.

3. **SIP Bridge / SIP Trunk** – This method is ideal for large implementations. Instead of just dumping all of the data to a mirror port, the recorder intelligently subscribes to the recorded devices. A simple example: if 1,000 devices exist on the network and you want to record 100 of them then it is ineffective to use the SIP SPAN method. The SIP Trunk method watches the 100 recorded devices and ignores the other 900 devices. This is much more efficient.

The last component of NG9-1-1 recording is used for data retrieval from the recording system and must be nonproprietary. To do this, the NG9-1-1 recorder must support RTSP (Real-Time Streaming Protocol) and web services allowing other equipment or users to subscribe and retrieve data. The good news about these three components is that you can share your data with others WITHOUT expensive, custom integration or other problems. Vendors can no longer hold your data hostage and charge you for it.

Traditional vs. NG9-1-1

As with any new technology, NG9-1-1 will take time to be fully implemented and adopted. Some questions to consider if you are in need of a recording system today and in the near future are:

1. What is the difference between traditional recording and NG9-1-1 recording?

2. Will the solution I buy today support both systems without any additional costs or forklift upgrades?

Let's explore the first question. The graph below gives a pictorial view of the differences between the Traditional 9-1-1 recording and NG9-1-1 recording.

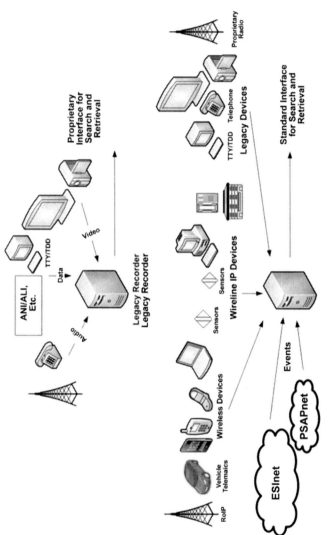

NG 9-1-1 Logging Service

33

The top of the graph shows a legacy recorder. A legacy recorder consists of:

1. Connects and records analog, digital, 911, and voice-over IP. Message types include voice. The voice comes from radio, 911, and telephones. TTY/TDD for the hearing impaired is also supported.
2. Basic data is available like ANI/ALI, radio ID, time/date, channel, and caller ID.
3. Basic search and retrieval, along with Live Recall, is standard with most traditional recorders.

The bottom of the graph shows an NG9-1-1 recorder. A NG9-1-1 recorder consists of:

1. SIP recording of all message types including voice, video, chat, text, and other NG data.
2. Logging Service to log all the interactions data associated with the event.
3. Standard search and retrieval interface.

You want to make sure that the recording system you purchase supports both of these environments—today and in the future. This is important even if you are three years out before NG is delivered to your center.

Let me explain what could happen if you don't do this. The new recording system you purchased does not support NG. You train your staff and pay money to have the system installed and running. If your agency keeps its recordings forever, then you keep your older system for data retrieval as well.

Fast-forward three years and you are in need of NG9-1-1 recording. The system you purchased does not support it and your sales representative suggests an "upgrade." This upgrade basically means pull the three-year-old recorder out and install a new one. With this mentality, you end up paying twice for a recording system that should service your needs for at least five to seven years. I am sure in this budget-tight economy, paying twice for something that should have been purchased once, will not be appreciated by the board or taxpayers.

Continuing with the hypothetical story … you now have three different systems in place. The first is the original recorder for playback only, the three-year-old recorder for playback, and now the NG recorder for current needs. And your staff needs to be RETRAINED on the NG recorder because the operation and architecture are different. A huge headache and waste of time, resources, and money that could have been avoided with smart planning.

In summary, you want to buy a recording system today that supports both traditional recording and NG9-1-1 recording in the current platform. **How do you guarantee this?** (This answer and a bit of advice will save your agency a ton of money. If you want, you can use some of your savings to purchase more copies of my book ☺.) What you do is get a letter *in writing* from the MANUFACTURER guaranteeing that there will be no platform change or forklift upgrade of your current system. Also, make sure the letter states that NG9-1-1 recording will be supported for no additional licensing or hardware costs for your agency. Also, if you are dealing with a reseller company, do NOT accept a letter from it. I am sure the reseller has good intentions and wants to protect you but resellers do NOT contractually bind the manufacturer—which is critical.

The last component I want to address is the radio system. As you know, the most expensive infrastructure component in 911 is the radio system. The standard interface for the radio system is known as the ISSI RoIP (Radio over IP) interface. ISSI is the accepted standard for NG9-1-1 radio communications and data sharing.

A short story to illustrate that inter-radio system communication is critical:

The terrorist attacks on September 11, 2001, were horrific events. Like all disasters, high stress showed the cracks in the system. When first responders from the various agencies rushed to Ground Zero in New York City, they did so with their respective equipment. Teams went into the buildings and saved lives. The problem occurred when the teams could NOT talk with each other. Imagine being 100 feet away in a disaster area and not being able to talk to the other team because they were on a different radio system. This was a problem then and it is still a problem more than ten years later.

The APCO Project 25 interface was designed to bridge this problem. It was created in the 1990s but adoption has taken time. APCO P25 allows for cross-radio system communication. P25 ISSI is a nonproprietary interface that enables RF subsystems built by different manufacturers to be connected together into wide-area networks. This provides extended coverage areas for subscriber units.

From an NG9-1-1 recording perspective, the ISSI RoIP interface allows for the recording of radio traffic in a nonproprietary fashion. This is another capability that is required of recorder manufacturers to support NG9-1-1.

What NG9-1-1 Recording is Not

NG9-1-1 is a hot topic in public safety and is the biggest change to happen in Dispatch Centers in the last thirty years. With so much hype, there are misconceptions. DSS has a large public safety community that we work with and some of the purchasing stories are horrific. I have received phone calls from high-level public safety officials asking me about our NG9-1-1 recording expertise. One gentleman was very upset on the phone until he recognized we were for real. I asked him why he was upset and he proceeded to tell me how vendors were using the term NG 9-1-1 to sell ANYTHING. The example he gave was a vendor selling NG9-1-1 chairs. Yes, chairs.

It is unfortunate that some vendors will say anything to get business. Let me clear up some of the confusion. Below is a list of features that are pitched as NG9-1-1 recording must-haves. Although they are good features, they have NOTHING to do with NG9-1-1 recording. If these are pitched to you as NG must-have features, proceed cautiously and contact NENA NG9-1-1 partner program directors at **http://www.nena.org** and ask for clarification.

1. **Screen Capture** – This is the ability to record the dispatcher's computer screen and play it back like a video. This is a great tool and enhances quality and training. (I recommend you buy it, but it has nothing to do with NG9-1-1 recording.)

2. **Workforce Optimization Solutions** – These are a suite of software applications that maximize

scheduling, training, and other analytics associated with Dispatch Center quality. These are excellent tools but they have nothing to do with NG9-1-1 recording capabilities.

3. **Mapping** – This feature allows you to plot and see location data in visual form. Mapping calls and incidents is an excellent feature and should be a part of your recording system. Vendors should include this at no extra charge. This is a great feature but has nothing to do with NG9-1-1 recording.

4. **Incident Recreation and Case Building** – Incident recreation allows you to recreate events and should be standard with any recording platform. The case-building functionality allows you to import other files, like PDF, Word documents, pictures, and video outside of the recording system to allow you to build a case for court and have the recordings and additional evidence together. Another great feature but it has nothing to do with NG9-1-1 recording.

In summary, be careful and do your research before drinking the vendor Kool-Aid. NG9-1-1 recording consists of three components: SIP recording, Logging Service, and RTSP retrieval. Anything else is simply vendor hype. To protect yourself, you can download **"9 NG9-1-1 Recording Questions You Should Ask Every Vendor"** at

http://www.dispatchimprovement.com/book/9-questions.aspx

3

NG Recording User Functionality

I n this section, I will discuss the benefits and feature sets required to attain the Holy Grail of Simplicity, Reliability, and Speed. The goal is to enhance your agency's quality initiatives as well as saving time and money.

Recording

Traditional recording-capture ties in all audio types, including radio, telephone, and 911. This audio can be captured in analog, digital, T1/E1, and VoIP formats. The recorders do this seamlessly in the same chassis. The recording platform should allow you to add additional communication types. If you want to capture email in your recording system, then you add an email-capture module allowing you to receive email from Windows Live, Microsoft Express, and other POP3/SMTP email providers.

The same holds true for premise-based video capture. If you want to add a few cameras to the recording system, then simply add a license for video capture. An example configuration is a 48-port audio recording system with three cameras that cover the jail cells and booking areas.

Capturing additional data types, like chat, sensors, and telematics should be included in the base system once your agency starts to receive this data. One way to insure that the recording system you purchase is ready for NG is to have these capture types presented to you live.

Questions to ask when investigating complete capture of all communication types TODAY:

1. Do you record analog, digital, T1/E1, VoIP, and SIP in the same system?

2. Do you require different hardware or software solutions for different capture types?

3. Can one solution record voice, email, chat, video, and NG data—or are multiple products required? (Note: you do not want to manage disparate products for this.)

4. Do you record email from Microsoft Exchange and other email formats? Can you show me an email in your system?

5. Do you record premise-video in your system? Can you show me a video in your system from a camera; not a computer screen? Note: Computer-screen capture and video are different functions.

Recording solutions must be integrated into one system. You want to manage one solution for all of your needs. Thus, one solution should record voice, video, computer screens, email, chat, and NG data. Avoid vendors that propose different products to accomplish recording.

Search

Most people have used Google. Google has changed the world. Think about it. You can search virtually any subject in Google and instantly receive a wealth of answers. Google search is a huge benefit and provides outstanding service. Best of all, it is free. If you look at the basic tenants of Google, it is fast, relevant, and even suggests what you might be looking for.

With technology like this, available to everybody including a five-year-old, why is recording technology still in the Dark Ages? Existing recorders today are pre-Google when it comes to search. You can only search on 5 percent of the repository contents, meaning you can find information searching by time/date, channel name, ANI/ALI, and phone number. If you are lucky, you can find recordings by Radio ID and alias as well.

When asked, how do you find your calls? this is the response heard all over the U.S.: *When there is an incident, we go to the CAD system and pull the incident and look at the time and date of when it happened. Once we know that, then we go to the recorder and punch in the time and the date and listen to the calls that come up. This usually takes about an hour or so to find the right calls.* This does not sound like a Google search to me.

A mandatory feature that your staff deserves is 100 percent content search. Your staff should be able to simply type in keywords, CAD incident numbers, or any other search phrase and find what they want, instantly. If you think about the other 95 percent of the NG recorders repository, it is filled with audio and text data. ALL OF THAT DATA NEEDS TO BE SEARCHABLE.

Finding all calls where "shots fired" is spoken is an example of 100 percent content search. Proactive search alerts you when "shots fired" or any other configured phrase is spoken. The recording system needs to be able to provide that functionality to you and your staff.

Everything with regard to the NG recorder needs to be proactive. Recorders are tools; not anchors. If you are looking to purchase a new system, you need to make sure 100 percent content search is part of it. Word of caution: most products on the market today DO NOT offer this functionality, so do your homework.

Another feature that is required to save your users a lot of time is relevance-based search results. This is especially true for large agencies. To cement this point, consider the following statistic: Google users perform BILLIONS of searches every day and 95 percent of them NEVER go to page two of the results. That figure illustrates the power of relevance-based search results. You should expect no less from a new recording system. Large agencies that record tens of thousands of calls per day need to have this functionality as standard.

Agencies have a wealth of information tied up in their host systems. A prime example is the CAD system. One thing that is critical is the ability to append CAD information to the recorded interactions without the need for expensive custom integrations. Tools exist today to simply get additional CAD-associated data and marry it to the recording system. Information can consist of anything that is important to you and your staff. Examples include CAD Incident number, call type, and call notes. There are others but you should be able to do this without a custom integration.

What is a custom integration and why is it bad? Custom integrations are when two vendors work together to make a "custom integration" between their two software platforms. The reason this is NOT the best solution is because custom integrations are expensive and not scalable. Let me give you an example to illustrate the point: Let's suppose you want to do a custom integration with your CAD system and your recorder (one that does not provide tools to do this without the integration). The backroom development boys for each company have to map out how they are going to do the integration. They do the work and you have your solution. You pay each company a lot of money for the work. You start to get the benefits of the integration and your CAD vendor has a new version it wants to roll out to you. Guess what? You get your new version and it breaks the integration. Now, you have to pay to have it fixed. This is why custom integrations between two companies can be a nightmare. In summary, you want to avoid custom integrations because of the high cost and headaches of maintenance.

As you can see, search functionality is critical for NG9-1-1 recording platforms. Realize that when your agency starts to accept NG9-1-1 data, the content bloat will increase by at least three times. You know the budget will not allow you to increase your staff by three times, so the tools you acquire need to be efficient and effective.

The 80/20 principle is effective here. You need the ability to find 80 percent of your interactions in 20 percent of the time it would normally take. This allows you and your staff to focus on Parkinson's Law and negate it. Parkinson's Law states: **"Work expands so as to fill the time available for its completion."** A simple example of this is a college term paper. Most college students end up writing it in the last week of the term but it took all term to complete. Since the content bloat of NG9-1-1 will increase three times, agencies cannot afford Parkinson's Law to take effect. Make sure the tools you invest in protect against this phenomenon.

Here are some questions you should ask potential recorder vendors:

1. How does your search work? Is it relevance-based? Show me.

2. Is your search engine full text searchable? If we are capturing email, chat, and other NG data, can we search *within* the text? Show me.

3. Is your search engine able to search for words and phrases inside the audio and video? If I wanted to find all the calls containing "shots fired," can I do this? Show me.

4. Can you populate the recording database with CAD data? How does your company do this? (If the answer is, "We have a custom integration for your agency" or if they expect you to write programing for it, don't buy it.)

Sharing

Sharing data is critical to Dispatch Centers but is also a double-edged sword. What do I mean? Dispatch Centers deal with life-and-death situations. Dispatchers are trained and conditioned to do so. Guess what? The public is NOT conditioned, so if information is shared that is NOT supposed to be shared then it can hurt the agency even though standard operating procedures were followed. Likewise, if information is withheld it is perceived that the agency is hiding something. This is especially true when FOIA requests come from attorneys. So, how do you share the data without compromising security? Let's find out.

Security

Security is a nebulous term that connotes several things. Get six IT guys in a room and you will have seven different security definitions and opinions. NG 9-1-1 recording systems contain a vast amount of data and access to this data is critical. You need to set up security to make sure that the right information is delivered to the right people at the right time. The system has to be flexible enough for full transparency. From a procedural standpoint, the agency needs to decide, based on responsibilities, which personnel have access to what. For example, dispatchers typically have access to their console position's data along with their own Quality Assessment information. Some agencies lock down this data in eight-hour increments to coincide with shift hours. Regardless of what channels, time, and data are shared, one thing is imperative and that is you need to have transparency in the system.

Transparency

The NG9-1-1 recording system needs to audit
EVERYTHING that happens in the system. You need to be
able to know who accessed what and what they did. Here are
examples of audited events:

1. John Smith listened to a 911 call on February 14,
   2011, at 1:10 a.m. You should simply be able to click
   on this log event and play that call.

2. Amy Apple redacted (blacked out) a 911 call on
   March 3, 2011, at 3:00 am. The call was downloaded
   and saved as redacted.

3. Jim Jones accessed live recall and flagged a radio
   transmission at 4:10 am.

Another critical component is user setup, which must be easy,
straightforward, and Active Directory (LDAP) compatible.
This is a technical term that I explore in detail in Appendix
A. This provides the following benefits to your agency:

1. Active Directory (LDAP) users and groups can be
   read and emulated in the NG9-1-1 recording system.
   This saves much setup time and when there is a
   change in the Active Directory it is automatically
   reflected in the recording system.

2. The users do NOT have to remember a separate user
   name and password for the recording system. Without
   this feature, it becomes a nightmare remembering
   ANOTHER user name and password. Dispatchers
   have enough to worry about, so the application needs
   to be flexible for them.

3. Single Sign On (SSO). If you are logged into your computer then the system automatically knows who you are and logs you in automatically.

Sharing Data

Now let's get into the good stuff: sharing data. First and foremost, do not let vendors hold your data hostage. You should be able to share your data and have as many users on the system as you want. You should not have to buy extra licenses to have multiple people access information. Likewise, you should not have different application software to access the system. This is a nightmare for IT and users. Remember, one browser-based application and unlimited users and you will save a fortune in time and money. To share data, you need several EASY and SECURE ways to do it.

1. **Links** – You need to share a reconstructed event with the first responders involved and other team members. Let's say the scenario consists of twenty recordings from 911, telephone, and radio transmissions. You want the ability to simply email a link to the people who need it. Links provide a significant time saver and are great for large scenarios where emailing these calls will NOT work because of the size. The last thing you want to do is email twenty recordings to thirty people. This will give your email system administrator a heart attack and eat up storage on the email system.

2. **Clipboard** – The Clipboard is an excellent feature that allows you to share data with people who are NOT configured users on the system. Basically, you

send a saved scenario to the Clipboard and designate it to be live for say seven days. The user that needs access to the data simply clicks the browser link and logs in in with the credentials providing a highly secure and audited way to share data. The Clipboard is powerful because the links have a time limit and expire, so you know the data is audited and not floating around somewhere on a disk.

3. **Any Device** –Ease of use is critical and people using iPads, iPhones, Android Tablets, Mobile Data Terminals, PCs and MACs need access. Accessing links from any of these devices anywhere is important. Seconds Save Lives and you should not be restricted to a particular device.

4. **Email** – Email functionality is standard from any recording system. Make sure all email events are audited for transparency. Email is handy when you crop a small segment of a call and send it to another user. Let's suppose there is a thirty-minute call and the meat of the call is one minute. You can simply crop the call and email it, thereby saving the recipient twenty-nine minutes of time.

5. **Save CD/DVD/USB** –You need the flexibility to save scenarios to external storage devices. Saving to CD/DVD/USB is standard on many systems. A free version of the recording application should be on the storage device so that the user simply clicks on the file and the application opens up, offering flexible playback features. The viewer works just like the main recording application and should be provided at no extra cost. Remember, it is your data and you

should never be charged to search, share, and report on it.

In summary, you want to make sure you have the flexibility to do whatever you want with YOUR data. Do not allow vendors to restrict you or charge you for access to the system. The goal is for you and your team to have an extremely flexible solution. Make sure that auditing and transparency are included so you know what is happening at all times.

Share Tools

Some additional tools are required and will save you and your team a lot of time. These tools are cropping, redacting, and altering.

1. **Redaction** – Remember the old days when you had to use a black marker to cross out information on paper? Redaction is the same thing. NG9-1-1 data needs redaction tools like blackout, highlight, and sticky notes. Anything you can do to paper, you can do on your NG data. NG data is more than just voice, so you need to be able to black out portions of recordings as well. If you have a FOIA request but there is privileged information that cannot be shared, then you use the redaction tool to put a tone on that part of the information. You can then save the redacted call and share it accordingly. Please note that redaction does NOT alter the original calls but simply creates a copy of it.

2. **Cropping** – Cropping allows you to take a slice of an audio or video file and save just that portion. If you have a long interaction but only need two minutes of

it, then you crop it and share that portion without altering the original.

3. **Altering** – Altering allows you to alter voices to hide identities. This is a new feature that you need to have on your system. Some states require this by law to hide the caller's identity and to encourage citizen autonomy. Altering will help agencies receive anonymous tips and catch bad guys. North Carolina adopted Senate bill 98 on June 27, 2011. If you would like to download the bill then please go to

http://www.ncleg.net/Sessions/2011/Bills/Senate/PDF/S98v1.pdf

Dispatch Improvement

Dispatch improvement is a framework to improve dispatch operations through training and tools. Seconds Save Lives and to improve on this, you must have the right tools and content available for your team.

Bottom line: agencies around the country perform quality differently. Some agencies are lights out in their passion for dispatch improvements and take it very seriously. Others have no clue, which is unfortunate. My goal is to help every center because public safety and dispatch improvement are critical for neighborhood awareness. Residents demand public safety. If you look at areas around the country that are growing, you will see that public safety is a critical component. Residents do not what to move into areas where they feel unsafe. Lousy public safety is a surefire way to lose tax revenue and residents. If the reputation of response times are bad then nine times out of ten the community is losing residents and tax revenue.

How do you improve dispatch operations and what tools are available?

There is a wealth of information to be reviewed, assessed, and analyzed from your NG9-1-1 recorder. The challenge is having the time to use it because budgets and staff are being cut.

Automated quality assessment starts with the right plumbing. The tools I will profile consist of Assessment Form Creation, Assessment Types, Reporting, Automating, and E-learning delivery. These tools are designed to save significant amounts of time and provide you trending data and feedback.

Assessment Forms

You need to craft objective assessment forms from the start. The assessment tool has to be flexible enough to handle any type of question—but objectivity is a key component. Question types include:

1. Yes / No

2. Yes / No / Not Applicable

3. Scale 1 to X

4. Scale – Strongly Agree to Strongly Disagree

5. Metrics – Metrics are section measures within the assessment itself. They allow for trending and improvements per dispatcher as well as the group.

Here are some sample questions from different assessment forms. For complete downloadable examples, visit: http://www.howtobuytechnology.com/QAForms

Call Intake Medical Assessment Form

Metrics:

1. CAD ENTRY

2. Location

3. MMR Transfer

4. Policies and Procedures

1. Verified incident address first?

☐ Yes   ☐ No   ☐ Obvious

2. Caller's name?

☐ Yes   ☐ No   ☐ N/A

3. Caller's address?

☐ Yes   ☐ No   ☐ N/A

4. Caller's phone number?

☐ Yes   ☐ No   ☐ N/A

5. Is patient breathing?

☐ Yes   ☐ No   ☐ Obvious

6. Is patient conscious?
    ☐ Yes   ☐ No   ☐ Obvious

7. Age/Sex of patient?
    ☐ Yes   ☐ No   ☐ N/A

8. Kept caller on the phone if necessary?
    ☐ Yes   ☐ No   ☐ N/A

9. Followed policy to dispatch first responders?
    ☐ Yes   ☐ No   ☐ N/A

10. Lengthy call time?
    ☐ Yes   ☐ No   ☐ N/A

11. Recognized and reacted to call appropriately?
    ☐ Yes   ☐ No   ☐ N/A

12. Was prepared to listen?
    ☐ Yes   ☐ No   ☐ N/A

13. Professional and courteous demeanor?
    ☐ Yes   ☐ No   ☐ N/A

14. Complete and accurate information entered?
    ☐ Yes   ☐ No

15. Call history, hot spot checked?
    ☐ Yes   ☐ No   ☐ N/A

16. Premise checked?

☐ Yes ☐ No ☐ N/A

17. Accurate address given to MMR?

☐ Yes ☐ No

18. Cross streets or common name used?

☐ Yes ☐ No

19. Township/city given?

☐ Yes ☐ No

20. Phone number given?

☐ Yes ☐ No

Other forms could include:

1. Call Intake Fire

2. Call Intake Law Enforcement

3. EMD

4. Other

This tool can be used in a number of ways. The benefits of putting your evaluations in the system include:

1. Centralized location for all assessment forms.

2. Reporting and trending over time to track improvements.

3. Multiple evaluations. The dispatch-team lead can evaluate and the dispatcher can self-evaluate. This

allows for flexible scoring and better training. The team lead and dispatcher can clarify any discrepancies and make improvements.

4. Assessments can be printed and signed off by both the dispatcher and team lead.

5. The assessments are tied to the event in the recording system so you have a true context of the interaction. You can hear the call and see what the dispatcher was doing on the screen along with reviewing the evaluation.

6. All notes associated with each question are saved with the evaluation form for later review.

Automated Search Functionality

One thing you want to avoid doing is manually looking for relevant calls to evaluate. Nobody has time to do this, especially dispatch supervisors. You want relevant calls queued automatically so you can simply review and score them WITHOUT having to manually find them. If you want to evaluate all calls that have a CAD incident number associated with them and a call type having to do with fire then those should automatically appear for your review. These automated tools are required in any good dispatch improvement system. Some of the tools include:

1. **Application Capture** allows you to set up automated searches from any data within the CAD system that is tied to the recording system.

2. **100% Content Search** allows you to perform automated searches for any content within the call that you want. For example, you can evaluate all calls with "shots fired" contained in the audio.

3. **Dashboard** is where your dispatch improvement calls are queued. You simply log into the system and your calls are delivered to you.

E-Learning Content Delivery

E-Learning is a method by which dispatchers can take computer-based training to enhance skill sets. Automating the delivery of the learning allows dispatchers to take the training and be quizzed at the end to test for competency. This is important and ties into Dispatch Center trending over time. Routing training to the dispatcher is an efficient way to make sure the training gets done and to audit the results.

Learning Styles

There are basically three learning styles: visual, auditory, and kinesthetic. Let's review each:

1. **Visual Learners**. Learn through seeing. These people see in pictures. They work best through displays, graphs, and other visual content. An easy way to identify visual learners is by using Google Maps. Do you read the directions or look at the picture of the map to find your destination? Visual learners like the map better than the step-by-step written directions. (An easy way to determine if people are visual is to listen to them talk. Typically you will hear phrases

like "I get the picture." "I can visualize that outcome." "I see what you mean." and "Looks good!")

2. **Auditory Learners**. Learn through listening. These people learn best through their ears. Lectures and learning through an iPOD or other recording device works great for auditory learners. Interpretation of communication has to do with tone, speed, pitch, and other nuances. Reading out loud is a helpful tool for these people. (An easy way to determine if people are auditory is to listen to them talk. Typically you will hear phrases like "I hear you." "That sounds good." and "I understand loud and clear.")

3. **Kinesthetic Learners**. Learn through moving, doing, and touching. These people use their bodies to learn. They think better by moving around and using their hands. They may even twirl their hair. (An easy way to determine if people are kinesthetic is to listen to them talk. Typically you will hear phrases like "It feels right." or "I have a good feeling.")

E-Learning can be designed in any way you see fit to best communicate the information. Thus, if a multi-media video file is created with a live call along with a movie, then this is delivering to two of the three learning types. You can also make the training interactive so kinesthetic learners are interacting with the lesson. These formats are powerful and will enhance dispatcher comprehension. Each training module can have a quiz to test retention at the end of the lesson.

In summary, E-learning is a great tool that each Dispatch Center needs to leverage. Automating the learning and content delivery is helpful based on the assessment results from the scoring initiatives discussed above. With these tools you can guarantee dispatch improvement, track the results, and see upward trends.

Dispatch Improvement Scorecard for Quality

Now that you have automated your dispatch quality, you can take it a step further and track the results by using the **Dispatch Improvement Scorecard**. This is a tool that allows each Dispatch Center to track the main pillars defined in its quality initiative. Before I dive into the details, let me provide a bit of history from the business world to show you the power of scorecards.

In Michael Gerber's book *E-Myth Revisited*, he chats about the power of creating systems and having people run those systems. Michael and his team studied the correlation of business failures and franchise successes for more than thirty years. The stats are pretty horrific. Fifty percent of businesses fail in the first five years with 50 percent of the remaining failing in the next five years. Thus 70 percent of businesses fail in ten years. On the flipside, 75 percent of franchises succeed in the same ten-year period. Looking at these stats begs several questions, but the most important are Why do franchises succeed? and What is the difference?

Franchises succeed because a detailed road map was created for the business owner to follow. The greatest franchise out there is McDonald's. When you think about it, Big Macs taste the same in Biloxi, Mississippi, as they do in Detroit, Michigan. McDonald's is one big system that can be run by average people. The great investor Warren Buffett always said that he'd much rather own a great business that could be run by average people than hard businesses that needed to be run by geniuses. This is the essence of why startup businesses fail and franchises succeed.

Are you wondering what does this have to do with Dispatch Improvement and scorecards? Systems in businesses are run by the numbers and the numbers are tracked by scorecards. The concept of the scorecard was created by Drs. Robert Kaplan and David Norton from Harvard Business School. Some of the greatest organizations in the world, like GE, use these tools to improve their businesses. Likewise, Dispatch Centers can use the Dispatch Improvement Scorecard to improve their operations with a much bigger payoff: Saving Lives.

The Dispatch Improvement Scorecard is a combination of number of calls taken per dispatcher, type of calls taken, average assessment scores before training, average assessment scores after training, and other ancillary data. For an in-depth look at an example scorecard, visit:

http://www.dispatchimprovement.com/book/scorecard.aspx

Dispatchers have to handle stress as well as plain, old public stupidity. Needless to say, patience and professionalism are required in ALL situations. Unfortunately, it only takes one screw-up to make the nightly news. In light of the tremendous workload, I decided to include a section detailing stupid 911 calls.

The first call is from a woman who is locked inside her car. The dispatcher was calm and professional enough to talk her into trying the device that opens the door. Guess what? The door opened! The dispatcher did not laugh or make jokes about the call. (I am sure she probably told everybody afterward but the good news is she did her job correctly.)

Another woman called 911 because her twelve-year-old daughter was out of control. She wanted the police to come to her house. The dispatcher made a joke and said, "Do you want us to come over and shoot her?" Obviously, he was joking but this simple comment ended up on Fox News. People need to understand 911 is designed for real emergencies.

This last call is unbelievable. A woman called 911 to complain that the Burger King she was at made her bacon cheeseburger wrong. She wanted a policeman to come down and protect her and make Burger King create the right burger for her.

I have great respect for dispatchers. I would love to hear about the funniest and oddest 911 calls you or your team has taken. I will protect the confidentiality of the stupid but would love to share in the laughs. You can post them on our blog site or email us directly with your stories.

http://blog.equature.com

4

Leadership

L eadership is essential to the success of any organization and it is imperative in building a great team. Setting up Dispatch Improvement programs and mentor programs are critical to reduce turnover and effectively make your Dispatch Center world-class. Let's look at business to show the power of leadership and then tie it into the **Dispatch Improvement Scorecard**.

Jim Collins wrote a book titled *Good to Great*. The concept is *good* is the enemy of *great* because of the comfort zone created by good. Jim and his team profiled highly successful companies that beat the market handily for fifteen years. He compared these companies with companies that were not able to achieve great status. There were several tenants that the successful companies showed in the research, but the one relevant here is the Level 5 Leader.

What is Level 5 Leadership?

Level 5 Leaders build enduring greatness through a paradoxical blend of personal humility and professional will. Let's compare two leaders and outline the differences. Lee Iacocca was a good leader and was instrumental in turning around Chrysler. He was an excellent Level 4 leader. Once Chrysler started to improve, Mr. Iacocca focused on himself, his book, and his popularity. Iacocca built Chrysler as a general in the army. The problem with this strategy is that when the General left, the army fell apart.

A Level 5 Leader is not centered. The Level 5 Leader has the organization and all stakeholders above his/her own self-interest. One of the goals of the Level 5 Leader is to build people stronger than him or herself. A great example is Ken Iverson from Nucor Steel. Iverson was a classic Level 5 Leader. He had the stakeholders (customers, employees, shareholders, and partners) all prioritized above himself. He built a wildly successful steel company in the 1980s. This was a huge task because overseas' competition was killing the big steel companies and U.S. Steel wanted government help. U.S. Steel executives were busy flying around in their corporate jets and furnishing their plush offices while Nucor was building a great company. Go to Google and search for Ken Iverson and Nucor Steel for more details. When Ken retired from Nucor, the company did not miss a beat because he built his leadership team. His ego was in check.

Dispatch Centers have a ton of moving parts and a strong team with a strong leader is required to deliver great service to your constituents.

What constitutes great leadership skills? For the sake of time, I will profile some of the work from John C. Maxwell. John has trained millions of leaders and is an authority on leadership. I will highlight some of his findings:

1. **The Law of Solid Ground** - Trust is the foundation of leadership. There is no two ways about it. You cannot build a billion dollar business over decades without trust. When you look at Apple, people trusted Steve Jobs. In contrast, think of Enron. Those executives built a house of cards. They hid their motives and lied to their employees. Once the trust was broken their careers ended. None of those executives could run another company again because they violated the Law of Solid Ground. It takes thirty years to build trust, integrity, and character—and only thirty seconds to lose it.

2. **The Law of Influence** – The true measure of leadership is influence–nothing more, nothing less. Think about this: Why would anybody retell history from 480 BC? The Spartan King Leonidas lead 300 Spartan soldiers into battle against the Persian army rumored to be in the millions. The Persian army was made of slaves while the Spartans were free men. The Law of Influence is seen in the fact that Xerxes, the Persian leader, would kill any of his men for victory and Leonidas would die for any of his men. Needless to say, the stand of the Spartans is still remembered as one of the greatest battles in history. All of the Spartans stayed and died because they were fighting for what they believed in and following a leader. That is Influence.

3. **Law of the Inner Circle** - The Law of the Inner Circle states the right people are your biggest asset. In other words, a leader's potential is determined by those closest to him. If you are just starting out in your career, then watch who you are working for. Where do they spend their time? With whom do they spend it? This is critical because the top five people you associate with on a regular basis determine where you are in life.

4. **The Law of Victory** - Leaders find ways for the team to win. Everybody knows that in business and war there is no silver medal. When Winston Churchill was asked what his aim was with regard to World War II, he replied, **"Victory. Victory at all costs, victory in spite of all terror, victory however long and hard the road may be; for without victory, there is no survival."**

These laws are important to building leadership skills. The effectiveness of your team is not linear but exponential in terms of effect. When you build leadership skills for yourself and your team then performance will improve.

Leadership Qualities

Let's examine some qualities of a good leader. (For more information on this topic, read *21 Qualities of a Leader* by John C. Maxwell.)

1. **Character** is best described with a story. Bill Lear created the Lear Jet. He was highly successful and a man of great character. He learned that three of his aircrafts crashed under mysterious circumstances. He

sent word to every customer and stopped shipping these planes until he could find and fix the problem. How did he do this? Here is the heart of the story: He flew the plane and recreated the problem by himself, putting his life on the line to get it fixed. He was willing to risk his success, his fortune, and even his life to solve the mystery of those crashes. He was not willing to sacrifice his character.

2. **Courage** is the ability to confront fear, pain, danger, and uncertainty and act rightly in the face of popular opposition. Eddie Rickenbacker set a world speed record at the Daytona 500, was an aerial combat pilot who recorded the most victories in World War I, survived a plane crash, and spent twenty-two days on a raft in the Pacific Ocean during World War II. When he was asked about his courage, he replied, "Courage is doing what you're afraid to do. There can be no courage unless you're scared."

3. **Discernment** is the act of determining the value of a certain subject or event. According to John Maxwell, "Smart leaders believe only half of what they hear. Discerning leaders know which half to believe." The Swiss had a monopoly on watches. One man had a digital design that he wanted to make. He took it to a company called Seiko. Needless to say, this changed the watch industry. One discerning decision can change your destiny.

4. **Listening** is critical in any endeavor. The leader who listens and engages the team will outperform the general with an army of pawns EVERY time. Listening is a whole-body experience. You need to

focus and dedicate yourself to this skill. Good listeners become great communicators. In Dale Carnegie's book *How to Win Friends and Influence People*, he profiled the art of listening and asking great questions. You cannot ask great questions if you don't listen and pay attention. A Cherokee saying states, **"Listen to the whispers and you won't have to hear the screams."**

Leadership is a lifelong study but it is worth the effort. The Dispatch Improvement Scorecard is designed to foster better service to your constituents, reduce staff turnover, and develop your people. Leadership skills are key components in achieving these goals.

5

Purchasing Methods

As you know, government agencies have guidelines for purchasing because they are spending taxpayer dollars. Unlike personal purchases or businesses, agencies always need to justify their expenditures because of this transparency. In this chapter I will discuss purchasing methods and options, along with the pros and cons of each.

Single Source Contracts

Single Source Contracts are a great way to purchase unique products and services assuming they enhance your center's quality of service. Again when it comes to NG9-1-1 recording, the goal is threefold: the platform needs to be simple, reliable, and fast because Seconds Save Lives. There are features in recording platforms that allow you to single source. The typical requirements for sole sourcing are:

1. Only one firm has a product that will meet the project's needs

2. Only one firm can do the work and the agency does not want multiple firms (i.e., manufacturer plus reseller)

3. Expert services are required and unique to the single firm

4. National security and/or public interest. For example, a U.S.-based manufacturer as opposed to a foreign one

The benefit to the agency is the speed of purchase. This is much easier and eliminates the wasted time associated with RFP's and bids.

Piggybacked Contracts

The goal of piggybacked contracts is to save the agency time and money by eliminating the duplication of work. If an agency you are familiar with has done its due diligence and has invested thousands of dollars in RFP/bid work, why not purchase that agency's results? Most organizations fail to think of this option, but with slashed budgets, this can be a significant money saver.

The pros for Piggybacked contracts are:

1. You do not have to duplicate the effort spent by the other agency.

2. You can contact the agency and discuss their after-purchase results. Are they happy with their choice?

3. You can review the summary and written recommendations and ask why the agency chose to purchase that particular system.

4. Save much time and money by leveraging OPE–other people's expertise.

Some of the drawbacks to piggybacked contracts are:

1. Do not buy old RFP results.

2. Make sure the agency you piggyback is similar to yours. Do not buy from an agency with a four-channel recorder when you need 300 channels.

3. Make sure the vendor the agency chose has performed. I know this seems intuitive but you want to verify this. Ronald Reagan used to say, "Trust but verify."

Negotiated Purchasing Contracts

General Services Agency (GSA) is a federal contract that allows you to buy equipment without spending a lot of time and money going out to RFP. Other contract examples are the Houston Galveston Area Council (HGAC) and CMAS, which is a California purchasing agreement. Other states differ and may have statewide purchasing agreements. Some of the benefits of these agreements are:

1. Your agency receives the pre-negotiated pricing based on a national (or other area-wide) purchasing agreement. If at all possible, purchase from GSA even for state contracts because pricing may be better.

2. You do not have to spend a lot of time, money, and resources sending out RFPs. (See costs in next section.)

3. Vendors that are on GSA are committed to the market. It is not an easy task for vendors to acquire contract status from GSA; so it shows commitment.

There is one drawback to using these contracts and that is you may have to pay to use them. However, the fee charged is minimal compared to what the bid process will cost you.

What is a sunset policy?

Sun setting is the concept where a manufacturer discontinues a platform. Most of you have probably received a letter that stated: "We are not going to support your system anymore." Pay us a bunch of money right now and we will give you a new one.

Sunset policies exist because most systems were created with a proprietary blend of hardware and software. Also, large manufacturers buy up smaller companies with no integration strategy and simply force customers to buy new systems. There are some major drawbacks to this approach.

If you consider document management, this industry has retention laws that state documents can NEVER be destroyed. You have to keep recordings FOREVER. For those of you unfamiliar with Document Management, it is a solution that converts paper documents into digital format. Now, imagine if every five years the system had to be changed out and the data was no longer available? Or worse, the product was SUN SETTED and you could no longer access your data? This is not a good way to do business.

To remedy this problem, NG recording systems need to be software-based and the architecture needs to be separate from the data model, meaning that regardless if the software is upgraded, the data is ALWAYS accessible. This eliminates the need to keep your old system online so you can access old data.

Recording retentions are different all over the country. Some agencies keep their recordings for thirty days; others keep it forever. The point is that the decision to sunset a product should be yours and NOT the manufacturer's.

Sunset Policy Review:

1. The manufacturer has a written policy and commitment to data compatibility regardless of the version of software. In other words, version 1.1 data should be readable ten years later by Version 5.2 software.

2. Make sure the system is *open architecture*. (I realize most vendors throw around this term.) Ask these three questions to protect yourself:

    i. **In what data format are the recordings, videos, email, text, and NG data stored**? They need to be open formats that can be played back and viewed with standard software. If you hear that they are *proprietary for security reasons*, do not buy the system. There are industry-standard ways to lock down data via security; proprietary formats are not best practices.

ii. **Can all the data be exported to an open format so you can leave your system and import your data elsewhere**? This is a critical question and separates the men from the boys. Confident partners have no problem with a policy like this because they know they can perform. If you get some form of "No" on this question, you do NOT want to work with that vendor. No vendor should hold your agency data-hostage.

iii. **Can the system be accessed from any device with proper security**? You should not have to install proprietary software to access the data. Data should be available real-time from any device, like an iPhone, iPad, Android Tablet, Android Smart Phone, Mobile data terminal, Windows-based computer, and Apple computers. All browsers like Firefox, Chrome, Safari, and Internet Explorer should work. Remember: Seconds Save Lives and if you cannot access your recordings in real time from anywhere it becomes useless.

Avoiding sunset policy vendors is critical for the Dispatch Center. This will protect your investment and be cost effective in the future. Also, it gives you control over your data and you will not be held hostage.

Manufacturer Purchase vs. Leasing

Some agencies have more flexibility purchasing items using their operating budget than their capital budget. Because of this, I will discuss some newer, more-prevalent options that some manufacturers offer directly to agencies. These total-solution bundles are treated as maintenance agreements and can offer a whole new system with full support for an annual payment. Please note, this is different than a lease.

Here is the skinny:

A lease is a contractual arrangement calling for the lessee (agency) to pay the lessor (owner or finance company) for the use of an asset. In the dispatch world a lease looks like this:

1. You decide to purchase a recording system from ABC Reseller.

2. You decide you want to lease the equipment; so ABC Reseller gives you the application and you send it to your attorney to review.

3. After all the paperwork and modifications are agreed upon by the Finance Company and the agency legal staff, you sign off.

4. ABC Reseller installs the recorder and you pay the finance company over X amount of years.

5. If the recorder needs service or maintenance you typically have to pay a separate agreement to ABC Reseller; unless if it is in the lease, then you pay interest on maintenance that you have not received yet.

6. Leasing companies charge higher rates on maintenance because there is no collateral and they are giving the bulk payment out to the reseller.

7. UFC form needs to be filled out declaring title on the equipment until it is paid off.

The benefit to leasing instead of purchasing is that the agency can pay for the recording system and maintenance without an upfront payment of cash. If the recorder can be acquired out of the operating budget then leasing may be the way to go— but there are some drawbacks to consider.

The main problem in leasing is the number of organizations involved in the transaction. You have a product made by a manufacturer, sold to you by a reseller, and owned by a finance company until you pay it off. If everything works well, no sweat; but what happens when there is a problem? Who is accountable? You may think the reseller is accountable but remember it received its money. If the reseller does not perform from a service standpoint, you still have to pay the finance company because it holds title to the equipment.

Thus, if you decide to withhold payments until the issues are resolved, the finance company can repossess the equipment and file a lien against the agency. The average recorder purchase in the U.S. is around $25,000. Having three organizations involved in this relatively small purchase is a waste of your agency's resources.

Again, leasing may make sense if you are purchasing a million dollar solution but not for such a small investment.

Manufacturer Maintenance Program

Recently in the recording market, some manufacturers are offering an exclusive maintenance program. These programs include:

1. A new recording system installed at your location

2. All maintenance and support included during the length of the agreement

3. All training included during the length of the agreement

4. Monthly or annual payment options to coincide with your operating budget cycle

The benefits of a manufacturer maintenance program are staggering because you are dealing with one company (not three) along with built in accountability. The recording manufacturer has to perform and provide service to your agency. If the manufacturer slips, then you have leverage with payment because the payments go to the manufacturer and not a finance company. Inherent in this program is the guarantee that I outlined earlier in the book. With this program you are dealing with one organization that can easily provide a guarantee if they are worth their weight and committed to the public safety market.

A manufacturer maintenance program differs from a lease program in three significant ways:

1. There is no need to file a UFC form because this is a maintenance program and not a lease.

2. There is no lengthy approval process with a third-party finance company.

3. In case of agency default, the manufacturer knows and understands the value of the equipment (a finance company does not). This means that the manufacturer will charge a lower interest rate than traditional leasing.

If you want more information on this type of program, visit:

http://www.dispatchimprovement.com/ppp.aspx

6

RFPs and Bids

RFPs and bids tend to take quite a bit of time. If you are new to purchasing equipment, then you will grow to hate this process. I realize that is a bold, negative statement but I am basing it on feedback from agencies over the last fifteen years. For the sake of brevity, I will outline the process and you can make your own determination.

Overview

Request for Proposals (RFP's) can be time consuming and expensive for both the vendors and even for the agency. The goal is to shed light on the true costs of RFPs in terms of length of time and financial cost. I will focus on government agencies doing RFPs for technology solutions. (In his book, *RFPs Suck*, Tom Searcy explains that everyone hates RFPs, including the agencies that create them.)Perceived Benefits

RFPs have benefits for projects over $150,000 in value. For projects below $150,000, the RFP process is burdensome and too costly to be effective. The main perceived benefit of the

RFP process is to reduce risks of the wrong solution. The concept of a lower price is another perceived benefit, but most agencies give up their negotiation power with the way they use and implement the RFP process.

The goals of the purchasing agency typically are:

1. Garner a solution to take care of the business issues defined for all stakeholders–end users, IT, and management.

2. Receive the best solution with the least Total Cost of Ownership and greatest value.

3. Eliminate purchasing risks from the wrong vendors and wrong solutions.

When these three criteria are met, then a successful solution is found and a win/win relationship is created between agency and vendor.

RFP Drawbacks

RFPs have several drawbacks above and beyond their expense. I will discuss the three main areas: lawsuit premium, inaccuracy premium, and inefficiency premium.

The *lawsuit premium* is the cost of avoiding a lawsuit by a participant challenging the accuracy and integrity of the selection process. Additional resources and expenses must be allocated when creating the RFP, including the legal review.

The *inaccuracy premium* has to do with the RFP process itself. Basically the agency puts out an RFP to solve a business problem. The issue with this is that most RFPs are written or copied from other sources that do not clearly define what the agency truly needs.

RFP motivations boil down to five uses: resolve political conflicts, mitigate low product expertise, substitute for purchasing expertise, leverage existing purchasing expertise, and preventing escalation of the original business problem. All of these prevent dialogue between buyer and seller, and they predefine not only the problem but much of the solution—which is the same as going to the doctor and telling her how to treat your illness.

The *inefficiency premium* is the premium an agency pays even though it states in most RFPs that the cost needs to be incurred by the responding vendor. Detailed below is a simple RFP timeline. (If you are new to purchasing, this process might seem daunting to you.)

1. Evaluate the Project (one to two months)

2. Plan and Document (one to three weeks)

3. Research and Target Vendors (one to three weeks)

4. Develop and Write RFP (one to two weeks)

5. Distribute RFP to Select Vendors (one to two weeks)

6. Allow Time for Vendors to Return Proposals (two to four weeks)

7. Evaluate Vendor Proposals (one to three weeks)

8. Compile a List of the Most Favorable Vendors (one to three weeks)

9. Select the Vendor (one day to a week)

10. Develop a Contract (two to four weeks)

Based on this ten-step process, it will take three to eight months to purchase your new system. Please see the enclosed spreadsheet to put a dollar amount on the RFP process. You can download the RFP cost calculator at

http://www.dispatchimprovement.com/rfp-calculator.aspx

Following is a visual example to give you an idea. For an eight-team evaluation committee to review proposals from six companies, the cost is $8,928. If you are buying a million dollar CAD system or radio system upgrade, then these costs are justified—but if you are purchasing a $35,000 NG9-1-1 recording system then it tends to be a waste of resources.

How much does it cost you to do an RFP for your 911 recorder?

Number of companies responding to RFP	6
Number of team members evaluating RFP	8
Average Hourly rate per team member	$23.25
Hours spent per employee on RFP	8
Total Cost of 911 Recorder RFP	$8,928.00

Assumptions:

Hourly Rate $ 23.25 Payscale.com

8 hours per employee spent on RFP SourceSolution.com

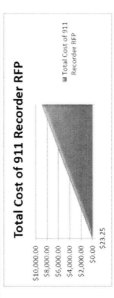

- Number of Companies responding to RFP
- Number of team members evaluating RFP
- Hours spent per employee on RFP

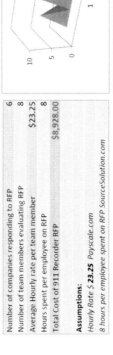

Total Cost of 911 Recorder RFP

- Total Cost of 911 Recorder RFP

7

Grants–Show Me the Money

I n this section, I will just touch on grants. This is a huge subject that is outside the scope of this book but my goal is to point you in the right direction to find money to purchase the NG9-1-1.

Basically, a grant is money given to an organization for a particular purpose. According to **www.Grants.gov**, grants are not benefits or entitlements. A federal grant is an award of financial assistance from a federal agency to a recipient to carry out a public purpose or support or stimulation authorized by a law of the United States. Federal grants are not federal assistance or loans to individuals. A federal grant may not be used to acquire property or services for the federal government's direct benefit.

Two departments to seek grants from are the Department of Justice (**http://www.justice.gov**) and Department of Homeland Security (**http://www.dhs.gov/index.shtm**). You can go **to www.Grants.gov** and search for Grant Opportunities.

After you find a potential source for money, how do you get it? Grant writing is a skill; there are professional grant writers. Depending on the amount of funds requested you might need to hire a professional. Bridget Newell, PhD, wrote an eight-page Best Practices Guide that is useful. The main highlights are:

1. Purpose of the Grant

2. Content

    a. Abstract or Summary

    b. Problem or Need Statement

    c. Solution or Scope

    d. Methods

    e. Benefits

    f. Qualifications

    g. Evaluation Plan

    h. Time Line

    i. Budget

    j. Conclusion

Dr. Newell also discusses writing techniques and other relevant information. The key here is to understand that your proposal will be considered against other proposals. Thus, following a logical, concise outline will increase your chances for successful funding. Visit **http://www.howtobuytechnology.com/grant** to download Dr. Newell's Best Practices Guide.

Appendix A

911 Jargon and Other Info

This information is to help you understand the intricacies of the recording market without the techno-babble. Some of these concepts are techy but I did my best to put real-world value on them from your point of view. When reading these questions, I want you to ask yourself, "Why is this important to me?"

1. What is a 911 recording system?

The 911 recording system records telephone and radio traffic into and out of your Dispatch Center. These systems started with the big open-reel tapes and are now computer-based. Most 911 centers use the system for liability purposes as well as to train their dispatchers.

2. What is a recording channel?

Each phone or radio position takes up a "channel" in the recording system. A channel can be a phone device, a trunk or a radio frequency, or a radio talk group.

3. What is 911 trunk-side recording?

Trunk-side recording is where the recording system records all activity on the trunks before the calls hit the phone system.

This is great for getting additional information. The benefit to the agency is that you get the on-hold activity as well as the pre-answer activity. What this means is that you can hear what the caller says BEFORE the dispatcher picks up the phone. Very beneficial! Some of our customers have prosecuted bad guys because of this configuration.

4. What is station/position recording?

The station/position recording is when "phone 2222" is on channel one in the recording system. This makes it easy to search the recording system because you know what position took the call. With 911 trunk-side recording you do NOT have this advantage because a call may come in on trunk 1 then the next call comes in on trunk 32.

5. Is it better to use just station-side recording and NOT trunk-side recording?

You should use a combination of the two on your 911 lines. Example: You configure the recording of the 911 trunks on a separate "channel card" in the recorder. This allows you to get all the on-hold talk activity as well as the pre-answer talk activity. You also configure the 911 positions on a different "channel card" in the recorder. This makes it easy to search for 911 calls by position. Thus you get the best of both worlds! You also get added redundancy because you are recording the 911 calls on two separate cards in the recording system. This is definitely the way to go and it should not cost much to do it this way. If budgets are tight, then you should record station-side only. This makes it easier to search calls and saves time.

6. What is a conventional radio system?

A conventional radio system is not trunked, so a conversation doesn't jump from frequency to frequency–two people must be tuned into the same frequency to talk with each other. From a recording standpoint, the radio system gives one audio output per frequency, which is connected to a recorder channel.

7. What is a trunked radio system?

Trunked radio systems use talk groups to utilize frequencies more efficiently. When you press the button to talk, the radio controller temporarily assigns you a frequency, and then releases it when you release the button. Anyone monitoring that talk group will hear you because all radios on that group will jump to that frequency. Since a conversation will jump from frequency to frequency, the recorder must follow the conversation by capturing the controller messages. This also allows you to search by RadioID, TalkGroup, or Alias (radio or talk group name). In the past, Motorola would provide LORI/LOMI cards to give the recorder one output per talk group, so capturing controller messages wasn't necessary. But, this was very expensive: you might have only ten frequencies, but sixty talk groups, so this method would require sixty recorder channels, plus the cost of the LORI/LOMI cards. Today, we record either the ten frequencies, or the consoles, or selected talk groups, then use the controller messages to follow the conversation and supply the additional search data. This is much more effective.

8. What is a P25 radio system?

Project 25 (P25 or APCO-25) refer to a suite of standards for digital radio communications for use by federal, state/province, and local public safety agencies in North

America to enable them to communicate with other agencies and mutual aid response teams in emergencies. The standard requires equipment from different manufacturers to be interoperable. In this regard, P25 fills the same role as the European Tetra protocol, although not interoperable with it. Modern recording systems must be P25 compliant because this is where the entire industry is going.

9. What is Next Generation 911 (NG9-1-1)?

For a great reference visit **http://www.its.dot.gov/ng911/index.htm**

In general NG9-1-1 will allow 911 Dispatch Centers to receive voice, text, and video from many devices. There are positive and negative feelings regarding NG9-1-1 because of the extra burden put on the agencies. 911 agencies today are already taxed and doing more with less.

10. Why should we record voice, email, and instant messaging?

As NG9-1-1 becomes more prevalent, Dispatch Centers will need to be able to record these communication types. A person might send a text message, perhaps with video, but there are actually several formats used to deliver that to you, including email. They might use this method because they're hearing impaired, or maybe there's been a shooting and they're hiding and unable to speak for fear of being discovered. If you are investing in a system, you do NOT want to buy a platform that does not support NG9-1-1.

11. How do we find calls quickly?

Agencies are taxed with doing more with less; thus it is imperative to be able to search and save calls ASAP. At a minimum, you should be able to search by time/date, channel, user, CLID, DTMF, ANI/ALI. With advanced systems, you can search by CLID Name, Radio ID, Talk Group, phrase search (in the call), or any combination based on relevance.

- CLID – Caller line Identification

- CLID Name – Caller line Identification Name

- DTMF – Dual-Tone Multi-Frequency (The phone number dialed out.)

- ANI/ALI – Automatic Number Identification/Automatic Location Identification

- RadioID – the numeric identifier of a specific radio on a trunked radio system

- Talk Group – a virtual group on which multiple radio users speak to each other on a trunked radio system

12. What is relevance search?

Enterprise Search engines like Google and Microsoft Live rank their searches based on relevance. Each search result is given a relevance score from highest to lowest. This is beneficial because it allows agencies to find their calls quickly and build more relevant searches.

13. Can you save calls and share them?

Yes. You should be able to save single recordings, multiple recordings, multiple recordings as a single file, and multiple recordings with all the data associated with them—and be able to share the data.

14. What is spoke time/date?

This is a feature of the recording system that allows you to put a voice that speaks the time and date of each call at the beginning of the calls. This is beneficial if you need to take the call to court.

15. What is FOIA?

Freedom of Information Act (FOIA) legislation, also called open records or (especially in the United States) sunshine laws, establish rules on access to information or records held by government bodies. In general, such laws define a legal process by which government information is required to be available to the public. These requests take a lot of time to fill for agencies; so the recording system must allow for easy use and quick search to save time. This is also referred as PITA (Pain in the Asterisk) by some agencies. These FOIA requests are time-sensitive so it is imperative to find the information quickly. All or most of the content delivered in the NG9-1-1 environment is expected to also be subject to FOIA.

16. What is Enterprise Search?

Enterprise Search is similar to Google and Microsoft Live Search. It utilizes the same advanced search technologies like relevance, operators, search builders, and browser technology to bring powerful results to end users. Recorders based on this model are ideal because of the ease of use and limited training required for agency staff.

17. What is screen recording?

Screen recording, or Screen Data Capture as it is known, is the method of recording the dispatcher's computer screens and aligning them with the voice calls. This is beneficial to verify data entry, identify training areas, and monitor overall quality of the Dispatch Center.

18. What is Digital Signature/Digital DataPrint?

Digital DataPrint is a software technique that authenticates and verifies recordings have not been tampered with. This is important to agencies that need to share the data in court.

19. What is Redaction?

Redaction is the method of "blacking out" certain portions of a recording. This is a useful feature because you can black out privileged information before sending the recording to the FOIA requester. Example: There is HIPPA information in the recording that can NOT be shared. You would simply redact the call, save it, then send it out. Old recording systems do not have this feature and require you to use a third-party application. Newer systems have the redaction capabilities built into the application.

Note: The Health Insurance Portability and Accountability Act (HIPAA) was enacted by the U.S. Congress in 1996. According to the Centers for Medicare and Medicaid Services (CMS) website, Title I of HIPAA protects health insurance coverage for workers and their families when they change or lose their jobs. Title II of HIPAA, known as the Administrative Simplification (AS) provisions, requires the establishment of national standards for electronic health care transactions and national identifiers for providers, health insurance plans and employers.

The Administration Simplification provisions also address the security and privacy of health data. The standards are meant to improve the efficiency and effectiveness of the nation's health care system by encouraging the widespread use of electronic data interchange in the U.S. health care system.

20. What is live monitor?

Live Monitor is a feature that allows you to listen to calls "as they happen" in your office. You can monitor one channel or multiple channels. This is beneficial if you have new dispatchers and you want to monitor them for training.

21. What is Instant Recall?

Instant Recall is a feature that allows you to pull back X minutes of audio instantly to verify information. This saves lives. The recorder protects your ASSets.

22. What is multi-channel playback?

Multi-channel playback is the method of playing multiple recordings from multiple channels simultaneously. It is used to give an accurate description of what happened at a point in time.

23. What is Scenario Reconstruction?

Scenario Reconstruction is multi-channel playback on steroids. It gives a graphical display of related calls and allows you to play them all back, or some of them back, based on your needs. You can also download the scenarios and email them. All of the call information can be viewed on the graph as well. Scenario Reconstruction is the quickest way to produce related calls and data in response to an official request. It's also the best way to get the whole picture of an incident for the purpose of review or post-incident assessment.

24. What is bookmarking?

Bookmarking is a feature that allows the end user to save searches and group the recordings based on specific needs. Thus you can save a group of recordings in the CASE 33434 file. This is similar to the Favorites settings in your Internet Explorer browser.

25. What is tagging?

Tagging allows end users to attach data that is relevant to the recordings. This can be a date/time, incident/case number, call type, or a description. Tags are searchable and displayed in columns for ease of use. A recording system should allow you to create your own tag fields and not limit the type or number that can be created.

26. What is sequential playback?

Sequential playback allows the end user to select calls and play them back in sequential order. This helps if you want to listen to calls exactly as they happened without having to hit the play button each time.

27. What is DVD/Tape archive?

The old recording systems archived recordings to DVD/Tape. As each storage medium improved, you typically needed to buy a new recording system to take advantage of it. The fundamental problem with this old method is that it takes time for the agencies to manage the archive media. Example: Sunday morning at 3:00 a.m. an alarm goes off because Side 2 of DVD 284 is full. Now the dispatcher has to call the supervisor to see if he can change the disk. This causes a lot of waste. Also, when disks are lost the data is gone as well.

The newer recording systems eliminate these housekeeping measures while keeping data safe and secure.

28. What is a Dashboard?

State-of-the-art recording systems have Dashboards. Dashboards are a landing page in the recording system that can be customized based on your job. It makes it easier for agency personnel to do their work. Dashboards can have parts that only help you with your daily functions.

29. What is SAN/NAS storage?

SAN stands for Storage Area Network and NAS stands for Network Attached Storage. Both formats provide agencies with additional storage and allows agencies to keep more data without the hassle of tapes or DVDs.

30. What is RAID storage?

RAID stands for Redundant Array of Inexpensive Disks. There are several RAID types, like RAID 1, 5, 10, 50, etc. The point is that it provides redundancy to your data. Typically you will want RAID 1 or 10. I would stay away from RAID 0 and RAID 5.

31. What is AD?

Active Directory (AD) is the directory service Microsoft provides you to manage users and devices on the network. AD handles users, groups, devices, login/logout, password rules, and security over the network. Your recording system needs to support Active Directory. The benefit to users is they do not have to remember another username and password for the system; they can simply use their Windows login account. It is also more secure than sending username and password data to the recorder across your network.

32. What is browser-based?

This means that the recording system uses Internet Explorer or Mozilla FireFox as the entry into the system. This is beneficial and saves a lot of time because you do NOT have to install any software on the computers you want to access the recording system. Also, this does NOT mean that your recorder is on the Internet. Some end users confuse browser-based with being on the Internet and that is not the case.

33. Can the recorder be accessed from anywhere?

Recording systems purchased today definitely should have the capability to be accessed from anywhere around the world SECURELY with no added software. With the newer platforms this is easy to do. The question is more of an agency procedure and not so much a technical question. The simple tech answer is yes but the agency may not want to allow it. You can use two techniques to accomplish this SSL and VPN.

34. What are SSL and VPN?

SSL stands for Secure Socket Layer. This is an encryption mechanism that allows for secure encrypted communications. If you look at your checking account online and see the little lock icon in the bottom right corner then it is using SSL to secure your session. This is one way to access the recording system from anywhere. VPN stands for Virtual Private Network. This is a technique that allows you to securely be on the network from anywhere. It provides secure remote access into the enterprise network.

35. What is an SQL database?

Older recording systems used proprietary databases to function. The problems with this were numerous: scalability, security, and interoperability with other technology. Structured Query Language (SQL) is an industry standard that most best-of-breed products use. Microsoft, IBM, and Oracle are premier database manufacturers with thousands of engineers that develop this software. It is much safer to use an industry standard instead of a proprietary database.

36. Why is an SQL database important to your agency?

SQL databases allow for easy data sharing among applications. Thus, if you want to run reports from CAD and the recorder to see what is going on, it is easy to do with an SQL database. Also, if you ever wanted to leave the recorder you purchased for a new one, it will be easy to import the data when the database is NOT proprietary. The big benefit for the agency is freedom of choice.

37. What is CAD?

CAD stands for Computer Aided Dispatch.

38. What is VoIP?

VoIP stands for Voice over Internet Protocol. All of the major vendors (Cisco, Microsoft, Positron, Motorola, etc.) have a VoIP offering in their newer equipment.

39. Can recorders record analog, digital, radio, T1, and VoIP within the same system?

The short answer is yes. All newer applications can do this. You should not invest in something that will need to be replaced simply because you've migrated from analog to digital or to VoIP from either.

40. What sort of security exists in best-of-breed recorders?

Best-of-breed recorders need to be compliant with Active Directory and support single sign-on. Also, recordings need to be secured so only authorized people can search and replay recordings. They also should support data encryption to prevent unauthorized access, and digital data prints on all recordings to verify the integrity of the data.

41. What are network shares?

Network shares are storage drives that are viewable on the network. Think of your F:\ drive on the network. That is a network share. Recorders must not use these because of security concerns. You do not want users to be able to browse the network and delete recordings. If the recorder you are looking at uses this architecture–RUN!

42. What is dispatch assessment?

Dispatch assessment is a module in recording systems that allows agencies to grade their dispatchers for quality. Forms can be set up and results can be reported on and trended over time. This is designed so the agency can improve its quality and reduce dispatcher turnover as well as identify training opportunities.

43. Why is assessment creation important?

Being a dispatcher is a high-pressure profession. The goal of assessments is to make everybody better and be able to share training data that is relevant for that goal. The more quality training for the dispatchers, the easier the job becomes over time. This could potentially save lives.

44. What do you recommend for creating assessments?

Assessment creation is a mix of art and science. In a nutshell, the assessments should be objective and not subjective. Yes/No answers are recommended because they are not subjective.

45. Why is it beneficial to use nonproprietary equipment?

Using nonproprietary equipment gives the agency flexibility if it wants to add storage or change things with regard to the recorder. If an agency is locked into a proprietary system, typically it can cost ten to twenty times more for certain repairs and equipment.

46. Do the recording systems have alarms in case they have a problem?

Yes. The typical alarms are: Recording/Not Recording, Running/Not Running, Channel Activity, Storage Low, and system restarted. There are additional alarm conditions that can be configured.

47. What is proactive alarming?

This means that your service provider is aware of an alarm condition when it happens. This provides for better support and can avoid major errors when minor errors are caught and fixed.

48. What constitutes good support?

This is a judgment call Industry standards are four-hour on-site response time, one-hour response for initial diagnosis, and proactive alarming with remote support.

49. What is free seating?

Free seating is the concept that dispatchers can sit anywhere in the center at any time. Thus, John may sit at position 1 today and at position 2 tomorrow.

50. What are some of the challenges of free seating?

In the old days, free seating was a challenge for Dispatch Assessment and finding calls. Typically you would have to listen to the call and then know it was Judy and do a manual assessment. The problem is you can NOT do any trend quality reporting for any random searches on Judy's calls unless you know where she sat every day. This wastes a lot of time in the Dispatch Center.

51. Can we solve our free-seating challenges?

Yes. Newer systems provide several ways to assign users and positions on the fly for free seating. The simplest way is to have the dispatcher login to an app to identify him or her which associates the user to a position. If the dispatchers login with unique logins then the recording system needs to be smart enough to know who is sitting where based on login. Both of these capabilities should be free.

52. Are there other free-seating solutions?

Yes. If there are third-party data streams with user/seating information then the recorder can use that information and assign seating automatically. Typically there is a charge for this type of free-seating integration.

53. Can you search by CAD incident number?

Yes. As long as that data is available, then the recorder can use it to associate the incident number to the call. This saves the agencies a lot of time because typically they search the CAD system for a time and date of the incident and then search the recorder. This is a two-step process which is very time consuming.

54. What is the NENA NG9-1-1 Partner Program?

This is a program where vendors work to provide interoperability to NG9-1-1 communications. As NG9-1-1 matures you will want to make sure that the recording solution you invest in is NG9-1-1 compliant.

55. How does the recorder connect to digital telephones?

Typically the phone vendor will break out each audio pair to a 66 block or 110 block five feet from the recording system. Then the audio pairs are cross-connected to the 66 or 110 block provided by the recording vendor. Thus, if there are ever any audio problems, it is easier to troubleshoot if the problem is with the recorder or the phones.

56. What is a 66 block?

A 66 block (also M-Block) is a type of punch down block used to connect sets of wires in a telephone system. 66 blocks are designed to terminate 22 through 26 AWG solid copper wire. The 25-pair standard non-split 66 Block contains fifty rows; each row has four columns of clips that are electrically bonded.

The 25-pair "Split 50" 66 Block is the industry standard for easy termination of voice cabling and is a standard network termination by telephone companies–generally on commercial properties. Each row contains four clips, but the left two clips are electrically isolated from the right two clips. 66 blocks pre-assembled with an RJ-21 female connector are available that accept a quick connection to a 25-pair cable with a male end. These connections are typically made between the block and the CPE (customer premise equipment).

57. What is a 110 block?

A 110 block is a type of punch down block used to connect sets of wires in a structured cabling system. 110 is also used to describe a type of Insulation-displacement connector used to terminate twisted-pair cables which use the same punch down tool as the 110 block. Usually 110 blocks are used in larger channel count installations.

58. How does the recorder connect to my analog telephone and radio lines?

Typically your phone/radio vendor will break out the lines that need to be recorded to a 66 or 110 block five feet from the recording system. This method is called *half-tapping*. Then the recorder is hooked to the block that is half-tapped.

59. What is half-tapping?

Half-tapping is the action of making analog trunks appear in two places for simultaneous service. Half-tapping refers to the duplication of service on the customer's side of the demarcation point. It's basically a "Y" connection. A demarcation point is the interconnection between the telephone company's communications facilities and the terminal equipment or wiring at a customer's premise.

60. What is the benefit of passively connecting to my telephone/radio equipment?

The main benefit of a passive connection is that if something happens to the recording equipment you do NOT take down the telephone, 911, or radio systems. In contrast, things that connect in a series often do NOT protect you this way. Thus, if there is a failure with a device in a series then all of the devices are affected. You want to make sure that the recording system you purchase is a passive system.

61. How does the recorder connect to my T1 or PRI?

Typically your phone vendor will provide a T Tap box that the recorder plugs into directly. This is a simple RJ45 cable that goes from the recorder to the T Tap box. It is important that this tap not bring down your circuit because of a recorder failure.

62. What is a T1?

A T1 is a digital transmission link that provides twenty-four voice channels. Each channel provides 64Kbps and the whole T1 provides 1.544Mbps of transmission capabilities. Agencies use T1s instead of analog lines because they are easier to work with and provide more channels in less space.

63. What is a PRI?

Primary Rate Interface (PRI) is the ISDN equivalent to a T1 circuit. The PRI provides 23B+D channels (B=Bearer channel, D=Data Channel). In easy terms this means that all the voice travels over twenty-three channels and all the signaling data travels on the D channel.

64. How does the recorder connect to record VoIP?

The phone recorder connects to a "Span or Mirror Port" on the network where the VoIP traffic exists. The connection utilizes a RJ45 cable. This is a standard network cable similar to the one your computer uses.

65. What is a span or mirror port?

Port mirroring is used on a network switch to send a copy of all network packets seen on one switch port (or an entire VLAN) to a network-monitoring connection on another switch port. This is commonly used for network appliances that require monitoring of network traffic, such as an intrusion-detection system or voice recorders. A VLAN(virtual LAN), is a group of hosts with a common set of requirements that communicate as if they were attached to the Broadcast domain, regardless of their physical location. A VLAN has the same attributes as a physical LAN, but it allows for end stations to be grouped together even if they are not located on the same network switch. Network reconfiguration can be done through software instead of physically relocating devices.

66. What is the difference between an NG9-1-1 Recorder and a traditional voice recorder?

While a voice recorder is only capable of recording audio, an NG9-1-1 recorder must be able to record voice, text (i.e., SMS text messages and email), pictures, and video (Department of Transportation Requirement Code SR-RCCAL-01-01). It must allow the user to search all of this content, regardless of type (FR-RCCAL-09-01). It must be capable of providing remote archive and access for all content and to correlate recordings of different media types to construct a single "recording set" (FR-RCCAL-02, FR-RCCAL-03, FR-RCCAL-10).

67. What types of communications must an NG9-1-1 Recorder capture?

Per the Department of Transportation Testing Requirements, an NG9-1-1 recorder must, at a minimum, be able to record voice, text (i.e., text messages and email), pictures, and video (Requirement Code SR-RCCAL-01-01). Other types of real-time data like alarms, telematics, and sensor data may also need to be captured (SR-RCCAL-01).

68. In NG9-1-1, what is considered a "call?"

In the NG9-1-1 definition, any real-time communication between a person needing assistance and a PSAP call taker is considered a call—whether voice, text, pictures, or video. The term *call* also includes "non-human-initiated" automatic events and alerts, such as alarms, telematics, and sensor data, which may also include real-time communications.

69. How many copies of an NG9-1-1 call must the recorder archive?

An NG9-1-1 Recorder must be capable of archiving both a local copy of the call (voice, text, pictures, video) and a remote copy of the same content. It must also make this content available for searching (Department of Transportation Requirements FR-RCCAL-02, FR-RCCAL-03).

70. What is "telematics"?

In the NG9-1-1 world, *telematics* refers to a system that is capable of two-way communication with a motor vehicle for the collection or transmission of information and commands. Vehicle systems from OnStar and ATX Group are telematics systems. They are capable of providing Advanced Automatic Collision Notification—data that is automatically transmitted by the vehicle in the event of a crash. The data includes speed and impact information, and is forwarded to the serving PSAP. This will save lives because it doesn't depend on action by the motorist, who may be severely injured or unconscious

71. Will NG9-1-1 replace the current 911 infrastructure?

Yes, in time the NG9-1-1 will replace current standards.

72. Who is driving NG9-1-1?

The U.S. Department of Transportation (USDOT) has been leading the initiative.

73. How long has NG9-1-1 been in development?

Planning for NG9-1-1 started in 2000 and was published in NENA's *Future Path Plan* in 2001.

74. What is the vision of NG9-1-1?

The stated goal of the USDOT project is: "To enable the general public to make a 9-1-1 'call' (any real-time communication–voice, text, or video) from any wired, wireless, or IP-based device, allowing the emergency services community to take advantage of advanced call delivery and other functions through new internetworking technologies based on open standards."

75. How can we pay for NG9-1-1?

The 911 Improvement Act of 2008 requires IP-enabled voice service providers to provide 9-1-1 service, allows state and tribal fees to pay for such services, and directs the Federal Communications Commission (FCC) to gather information to facilitate these services. The Act also provides for grants to public agencies, and requires the E-911 Implementation Coordination Office to develop a national plan for migrating to a national IP-enabled emergency network.

76. Who are the major stakeholders for NG9-1-1?

The major stakeholders are State and Local 911 agencies, public safety and emergency management agencies, and federal departments (Transportation, Homeland Security. and FCC).

77. Who are the major contributors for the NG9-1-1 standards?

The major contributors are NENA, APCO, IETF (Internet Engineering Task Force), and TIA (Telecommunications Industry Association).

78. What is SIP?

SIP stands for Session Initiation Protocol and is used for data delivery.

79. How will NG9-1-1 data be delivered to the PSAP?

Content comes in to the PSAP over SIP – used for years to carry VoIP, but capable of carrying any type of data.

80. When I transfer a call from one agency to another, I lose all the associated call information. Is that the same under NG9-1-1?

No. A PSAP can transfer a call to another agency, along with all data associated with it.

81. Will the dispatcher be able to share data (pictures, video, etc.) with the first responders under NG9-1-1?

Yes. Dispatchers can forward needed data to responders, including pictures, video, medical, or supplementary data.

82. Will vendors have to work together under NG9-1-1?

No. There are many misconceptions about this in the market place. NG9-1-1 requires interoperability based on standards. In order for vendors to be NG9-1-1 compliant, they have to follow the standards. This is good news because proprietary vendor relationships are no longer required for better functionality. This will save PSAPs money.

83. Will systems work together under NG9-1-1?

Yes. NG standards allow systems from different vendors to interoperate "right out of the box."

84. Can dispatchers work remotely under NG9-1-1?

Yes. Under NG9-1-1, dispatchers will be able to connect to systems from anywhere and work remotely. This may help Dispatch Centers with staffing constraints. We are entering a world where "virtual dispatchers" are a reality.

85. Must all equipment be onsite under NG9-1-1?

No. Equipment can be anywhere on the network.

86. If my PSAP does a consolidation with other PSAPs, can we share the equipment?

Yes. Agencies can team up and purchase equipment that is shared in the "Cloud." The benefit of this is scalability and resilience of equipment.

87. Does my equipment have to be offsite under NG9-1-1?

No. Your equipment can be deployed on premise just like it is today. Having your equipment located offsite or onsite is a preference of the agency; not a legal mandate.

88. How can we consolidate to save money?

NG9-1-1 allows you to easily consolidate and share systems as "services" with other jurisdictions. This provides greater functionality at a lower cost.

89. How do we cover NG9-1-1 transition costs?

There are a couple of ways to do this. Congress provides multiple grant programs that provide funding, and APCO & NENA provide information and guidance.

90. What do you recommend for writing grants?

I suggest you do the following:

- Start by surveying what you have

- Map out what you need to add to support NG9-1-1

- Create a transition plan

- Ask vendors for input and others at 911talk@listserv.nena.org

- Write your grant proposal(s) from your real plan, using real numbers provided by vendors

- If you want more information, contact me because we have worked with other agencies regarding project plans

Appendix B

Sample Money-Back Guarantee

The focal point of a Money-Back Guarantee is the amount of time you have AFTER acceptance to return the equipment and the amount of the return. Remember, this is designed to put the risk where it should be. The risk needs to be on the vendor you partner with and NOT your agency.

Also, you should not have to ask for this document. The vendors you are considering should provide this as standard protocol. If you have to ask for it, then you need to be cautious because that means the vendor does not typically offer it.

110% Money-Back Satisfaction Guarantee

"ABC Company" is pleased to offer this Money-Back Satisfaction Guarantee. As a manufacturer and developer of Next Generation 9-1-1 Recording Solutions, we are in direct contact with our customers. We have over "X years" experience in servicing the Public Safety community and understand the needs and challenges you face each day. We have a long track record of success which allows us to offer the following guarantee:

Within 6 (six) months after system acceptance, in the event the NG9-1-1 Recording system does not perform to standard 911 recording features and functions then "YOUR AGENCY" can terminate the agreement with 90 (ninety) days' notice to correct the issues and receive a full refund plus 10%. We respect your time and will not waste it. We look forward to creating a long-term business partnership.

ABC COMPANY   YOUR AGENCY

By:_____   By:_____
Print Name:_____   Print Name:_____
Date:_____   Date:_____

Appendix C

Sample Dispatch Improvement Scorecard

The Dispatch Improvement Scorecard is designed to help your agency stay on track and improve Dispatch Operations. This sample scorecard below provides a means to measure your progress being made as you implement new training initiatives.

Dispatch Improvement Score Card
Cummulative All Dispatchers

	Actual Assessments Taken	Plan assessments taken	Difference	% to plan	Actual Score All Metrics	Target Score All Metrics	% difference to plan	Actual E-learning taken	Plan E-learning taken	Difference	% to plan
Jan	80	100	-20	80.00%	70.00%	100.00%	-30.00%	5	10	-5	50.00%
Feb	105	100	5	105.00%	80.00%	100.00%	-20.00%	6	10	-4	60.00%
March	75	100	-25	75.00%	75.00%	100.00%	-25.00%	4	10	-6	40.00%
April	90	100	-10	90.00%	76.00%	100.00%	-24.00%	7	10	-3	70.00%
May	110	100	10	110.00%	90.00%	100.00%	-10.00%	8	10	-2	80.00%
June	110	100	10	110.00%	89.00%	100.00%	-11.00%	9	10	-1	90.00%
July	105	100	5	105.00%	67.00%	100.00%	-33.00%	11	10	1	110.00%
Aug	118	100	18	118.00%	77.00%	100.00%	-23.00%	11	10	1	110.00%
Sep	80	100	-20	80.00%	87.00%	100.00%	-13.00%	13	10	3	130.00%
Oct	75	100	-25	75.00%	76.00%	100.00%	-24.00%	10	10	0	100.00%
Nov	90	100	-10	90.00%	92.00%	100.00%	-8.00%	8	10	-2	80.00%
Dec	83	100	-17	83.00%	96.00%	100.00%	-4.00%	8	10	-2	80.00%
total	1121	1200	-79	93.42%	81.25%	100.00%	-18.75%	100	120	-20	83.33%

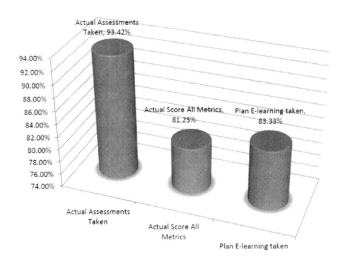

Actual Score All Metrics %

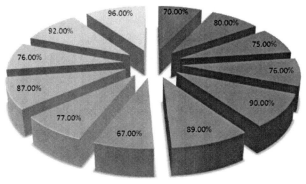

🞕 Jan   🞕 Feb   🞕 March   🞕 April   🞕 May   🞕 June   🞕 July   🞕 Aug   🞕 Sep   🞕 Oct   🞕 Nov   🞕 Dec

Actual Assesments Difference %

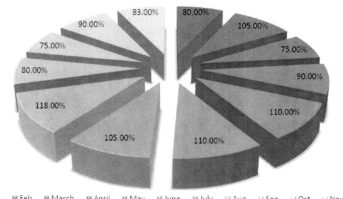

Jan Feb March April May June July Aug Sep Oct Nov Dec

E-learning taken difference %

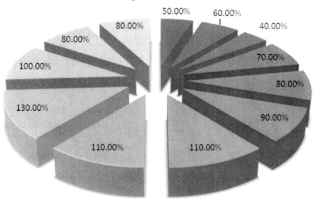

Jan Feb March April May June July Aug Sep Oct Nov Dec

Index

CPSIA information can be obtained at www.ICGtesting.com
Printed in the USA
BVOW01s1609230913

331875BV00003B/7/P